WHAT TO DO IF THE MIND DOES NOT DEVELOP

WHAT TO DO IF THE MIND DOES NOT DEVELOP

A Psychoanalytic Study of Pervasive Developmental Disorders

Roberto Bertolini

Routledge
Taylor & Francis Group
LONDON AND NEW YORK

Originally published in Italian as *Che fare se la mente non nasce: Uno studio psicoanalitico dei disturbi pervasivi dello sviluppo* by Bruno Mondadori in 2015.

First published 2017 by Karnac Books Ltd.

2 Park Square, Milton Park, Abingdon, Oxfordshire OX14 4RN
52 Vanderbilt Avenue, New York, NY 10017

Routledge is an imprint of the Taylor & Francis Group, an informa business

First issued in hardback 2019

Translated by Aldo Grassi

British Library Cataloguing in Publication Data

A C.I.P. for this book is available from the British Library

ISBN-13: 978-1-78220-403-9 (pbk)
ISBN-13: 978-0-367-32971-6 (hbk)

Typeset by Medlar Publishing Solutions Pvt Ltd, India

To Ornella, my life companion

CONTENTS

ACKNOWLEDGEMENTS

There are many people to whom I am grateful for assisting me in the writing of this book.

First of all I would like to thank Pearson, my publisher in Italy, for publishing the Italian version of this book in the University Series of Bruno Mondadori (2015) and the publishers of *Richard & Piggle*, Pensiero Scientifico, for the Italian version of Chapter Four (1996) of which I am the copyright holder.

I am also grateful to the following psychotherapists for their permission to use material from their patients' sessions, infant observations or conference records: Simonetta Lunati in Chapter Two (Carlotta), Ornella Caccia (Vittorio) and Susanna Maiello Hunzigher (Antonio) in Chapter Four, and Serena Latmiral in Chapter Three ("the little rascal") and Associazione Culturale Racker from Venice in Chapter Five (initial quotation).

Then I would like to thank Harper Collins Publisher for the written permission to reprint in Chapter Three the excerpts of copyrighted material from pages 22–26 of *The Blue Bear* by Lynn Schooler, and Ornella Caccia for verbal permission to quote in Chapter Five excerpts from "Differences between primitive and psychotic aspects in infant mental development", a paper first published in Italian (2012) by Pensiero

Scientifico Editore, and translated into English for this edition for the first time.

Lastly I would like to express my gratitude to Karnac books for agreeing to publish the English version of this book and to those people who assisted me in its editing: Oliver Rathbone, Cecily Blench, Constance Govindin, Kate Pearce, Martin Pettitt, and Rod Tweedy.

ABOUT THE AUTHOR

Roberto Bertolini has a degree in medicine; he specialised in neurology at the Catholic University in Rome and in child psychotherapy at the Tavistock Clinic in London, where he was for many years a visiting teacher for the program, "Work with disruptive adolescents".

He is a teacher of the scuola quadriennale in child psychotherapy at the Centro Studi Martha Harris in Florence and tutor of the Tavistock model courses in observational studies and child mental health in italy.

He conducts training and clinical supervision for mental health and social services professionals in Italy and abroad. He is the author of books and articles on child development and primitive psychopathology.

PREFACE

Dr Alberto Hahn

Reading this book has provided a much-needed injection of faith in the future of our discipline, and it is well known how scarce this opportunity has become at a time when psychoanalytical thinking has been transformed into something that frequently departs from what our teachers in the sixties and seventies of the twentieth century conveyed through their admirable inspiration and sensitivity, so that at times the core values of psychoanalysis become unrecognisable.

It is therefore very satisfying to read, in this volume, accounts of clinical work with children at the more disturbed end of the pathological spectrum with a pervasive disturbance in their development, in particular the delicate and detailed observations of the transference situations. These alone should make this a text-book for new generations of child psychotherapists and analysts as it emphasises the importance of minute and thorough clinical observation. We should regard this as the main ingredient for thinking and understanding our patients and our own states of mind, and for the way in which it enriches not only our capacity for empathy but also allows us to develop a theoretical compass that is based on our personal experience of the transference and countertransference.

Donald Meltzer's contribution to the understanding of autism and post autistic states is the backdrop to this work and it is Bertolini's contribution that occupies a prominent and insightful place here among the authors who specialise in working with children with these pathologies.

Bertolini clearly shows us in this book that there are increasing layers that different patients and their idiosyncratic transferences add to the overall clinical picture of a) what is the experience they have of themselves, b) the nature of psychic pain, c) of how we can help them, how we think, how we talk and what we do or not do, and d) what is the price we pay for undertaking this challenge, as is clearly stated in Chapter Nine.

Like the above, this volume encompasses an impressive body of knowledge that has been accumulated throughout the author's life and is didactic, consistent, articulate, sensitive, and intelligent. The consistency and sensitivity are shown in the work done in the seventies and eighties as in Chapter Seven and is followed through in later papers and one can see the evolution of his thinking and its originality and creativity.

As with all inspiring works, our attention is drawn to some basic issues which will be familiar to anybody who works analytically with these children: the different quality and intensity of pain as expressed in the transference, the importance of recognising that which promotes development rather than only that which impedes it, the importance of the countertransference in the receptivity of unconscious communications, the special language required for each patient rather than the trite repetition of well-rehearsed "wisdom" where the link to the patient takes second place to the "wondrous" interpretation centred activity of the (narcissistic unthinking) analyst.

In other words, it is written for people we assume recognise the analytic language we use. In consideration to a readership that comes from different backgrounds, simple definitions of technical terms are interspersed in the clinical notes and the appendixes (such as projective identification, autistic disturbance or the claustrum).

I believe that it is ideas, like the ones Bertolini develops in this text that provoke us and have a capacity to foster a turbulence that stimulates our questioning, our curiosity and our thinking ability. A multitude of ideas stand out for this reader and only using this space for a brief discussion of some of them can do them justice. Think of the following paragraphs as a psychoanalytic "*amuse bouche*".

Chapter Three, written in 2006, benefits from a brief introduction which comes across as a lucid description of the author's own sources of imaginative stimulation, as he also does later in the book regarding Goldilocks, Pinocchio, Giacometti, dendrochronology, etc. It means that if one is so disposed, these patients offer us opportunities for inspiration—as all patients actually do, something we frequently fail to convey to our students. Apropos this subject, "closing off" and dreaming in the presence of patient Rebecca is something that might be cross referenced with Donald Meltzer's writing on counter-dreaming and its relation to intuition.

In the discussion of fourteen-year-old A, in Chapter Four, the patient is described, almost in passing, "like a drunkard". This observation encapsulates a view in which we might be able to think about a state not unlike intoxication of the mind that prevents attention to remain in any place for any length of time. This results in his fidgety attention manically jumping from one object (or fragment of an object) to another, aborting in the process the emergence of emotionality.

The theme of the disruption of emotionality is repeated in some of the other patients where the author describes links, like joints, that are attacked in the mind and sabotage the capacity for introjection of the analytic containing function. It may be that it is this manic "jumping about" alternating with the collapse of depression—rather than the actual emotional contact as is suggested—which promotes a state of mind that overrides a precarious containing capacity which leads to disintegration. The absence of emotional links does not attract destructive attacks and the manic depressive conjunction itself encourages an avoidance of emotionality. This solves—for the time being—the dread of a breakdown as emotions, felt to be intrinsically painful act like antibodies in an autoimmune system by turning against the possibility of integration and the self.

In the case of T in Chapter Six, Bertolini questions if the painful acknowledgement of dependence is responsible for a psychological disaster that leads to the dismantling of the psychic apparatus. I thought that perhaps the retreat from pain was a retreat from contact and involvement due to the "lethal impact" as he rightly calls it, of the toxicity created by poisonous projections into the dependency link.

Chapter Nine is the most personal and highlights the importance of countertransference awareness. This links, almost "obviously", with the work of Dario Sor, an Argentinian psychoanalyst, a sensitive and intuitive clinician, and a Bion scholar who wrote a book on the subject of "*El darse cuenta*" (on becoming aware). One last thought regarding the examination of the countertransference. I do think that the area that is perhaps most productive is the one that lays bare our ignorance and confusion and yet allows us to keep thinking and conceptualising our experience on the patient's behalf. Clearly, it is not the patient who has to follow the route that goes from having a vision (inspired by wishful thinking perhaps) to the recognition of a presence (in terms of mental or sensorial apprehension). This spectrum of internal reality that we cover in our analytic work (in particular with patients who are on the autistic/psychotic spectrum with serious developmental damage, but not only) does eventually lead to the creation of meaning that brings sustenance and nurtures both the patient and analyst. It helps us in our effort to remain actively interested and attentive and it is of great value to the patient where there is some sense of awareness of positive attributes of internal objects, i.e., when they reach a position in which they can internalise the experience of goodness as a mitigating factor of the psychotic disaster they are trying to recover from.

Also, I am not sure I think of the pathological countertransference as "pathological". What Bertolini describes is a series of successes and failures in empathy due to heavy contamination of a pathological field—what he called "negative contagion"—a very timely oxymoron.

Matching our responsive countertransference to a disturbed (sometimes delirious) transference does not make our response pathological although it can be bizarre, difficult to recognise, weakening, and sometimes bound to be evacuated through acting out. This difficulty to recognise contain and live with this counter transference is what I would call work. Perhaps the "pathological" label should remain a subjective factor to be discussed in another context.

The reader will have seen how easy it is to become very involved in thinking about these matters and how great the temptation is to perpetuate this dialogue into what makes our work so interesting. This alone is a tribute to this book, which conveys the author's most convincing passionate statement about the healthy survival of good analytic practice.

A real treat lies ahead for the reader …

PROLOGUE

> No: it is not yours to open buds into blossoms.
> Shake the bud, strike it;
> it is beyond your power to make it blossom.
> Your touch soils it,
> you tear its petals to pieces
> and strew them in the dust.
> But no colours appear, and no perfume.
> Ah! It is not for you to open the bud into a blossom.
> [...]
> Tagore, R. (1916, p. XVIII)

In this book I will recount my clinical experience with children and adolescents suffering from pervasive developmental disorders, something that I have been able to learn in my work as a child therapist or supervisor in the course of about thirty years.

My interest in this type of psychopathology was born when I was still a young doctor. Towards the end of the 1960s, for the first time in my professional life I had the chance to observe, from behind a one-way mirror at the Institute of Psychology of the Department of Medicine and Surgery of the Catholic University of the Sacred Heart of Rome (UCSC) where I studied and worked, a few sessions of psychotherapy with an autistic child conducted by Dr Salomon Resnik. I remember that on such an occasion I made some important discoveries. First of all, I realised that it was possible to resist the apparent indifference of an autistic child and the sense of alienation that his mysterious and somewhat bizarre behaviour generated in an intersubjective relationship, thus managing to approach him and to establish some contact with his way of being in the world.

At the same time I became immediately aware that, in order to achieve this result, the therapist needed to be able to use his or her attention in an empathic and imaginative manner.

Dr Resnik made me understand how his therapeutic approach was supported by his great aesthetic sensitivity. I noticed that, at a certain moment, he would approach the body, the face, the movements of his young patient; the following moment he would move away, most delicately, never losing sight of him. In this alternation of movements, to and fro, he imperceptibly but repeatedly invited his patient to do the same with him, without ever forcing him one way or another. I thought I was witnessing a dance in which one dancer was trying to find a common rhythm with his partner or a shape that might represent both; or the experience of a visitor at an art exhibition who, facing the apparently incomprehensible and mysterious work of a surrealist or abstract painter, instead of running away, makes several attempts with his eyes to find something that might help him make sense of the painting in front of him, through a study of its compositional aspects, trusting that he will eventually make some interesting discoveries.

Then, a few years later, while I was attending the specialist course in Neurology in the same Department of Medicine and Surgery, I noticed how "beautiful" an autistic boy was. This discovery made me increasingly aware of the tragedy of such a psychopathological condition in which what creates contiguity, interest, intimacy, appeal, and attraction, namely beauty, harmony of movement, order, colour, and song, remained impervious to any communicative and social intentionality and was instead trapped into an unfathomable solipsism.

In the course of a consultation in the paediatric ward of Agostino Gemelli University Hospital in Rome, I was able to observe a young boy of four or five years old, with extremely beautiful features, harmonious in his movements, who was completely lost in his dances, the fluttering of his hands, his endlessly repeated melodious chant. The first thing I thought when I met him was that when he was born he had suffered from a sort of intolerable disappointment, and that he was now punishing us: "What, or who, could have betrayed his expectations in such a painful way?" This was an impression that I then found in my work with other patients similar to him. His repeated dance-like gestures had seemed to me like the representation of a heroic, stubborn, relentless attempt "to be there", through the sensual possession of the shapes, motions, colours, and surfaces of everything that was within his reach.

Finally, there is a clinical experience in the period of my medical training that left a deep mark in my way of thinking about the psychic life of children, which is very likely to have determined my choice of becoming a child psychoanalyst. This experience is linked to my meeting with a young patient of seven or eight years of age who was suffering from a serious degenerative illness of the central nervous system and was hospitalised in the clinic for nervous and mental illnesses where I worked as a young trainee in neurology. In only a few months he had helplessly experienced a progressive decline in his motor and intellective skills and had become increasingly less autonomous, also because of epileptic crises, which could not be cured by means of commonly used medications. To my great surprise, he developed an intense attachment and a deep liking towards me. In his lucid moments he asked his parents to take him to the medical room where I worked, because he wanted to talk to me about the notebooks and textbooks that he had left at home; and on the day he was going to be discharged (not because he had recovered, but so that he could die at home in his bed), he told me that he would come back here to see me and show me his homework, so that I could understand how good and diligent he was in reading and writing.

I remember that in response to his attachment I developed a particular attention towards him, learning to keep him in my mind in a unique and complex way, which helped me to look after him better, and to acknowledge his clinical condition with more accuracy. On a few occasions, this allowed me to be quite timely in administering the proper medication, so that an epileptic fit did not evolve in a malignant epileptic state. Thus, for the first time, I discovered the mysterious phenomenon of infantile transference, of empathic identification: that aspect of human communication that makes it possible for normally capable children, even in extreme situations like the one I have just described, to arouse in the adult caregiver a particular maternal or paternal attention, which is helpful to their physical and mental development. At the same time, however, I became even more painfully aware that there are children, even "beautiful" ones, who are unable—unlike my neurological patient—to seek and establish a passionate relationship with another person.

The contents of this book, however, illustrate what happened later, during and after my training in psychoanalytic psychotherapy for children at the Tavistock Clinic in London. That was a period in my professional life during which I was fortunate enough to personally see—without any traumatic interruption, and for several years—a number of children and adolescents who had a diagnosis of pervasive developmental disorder. It was certainly a limited number of cases—seven altogether—but I still have detailed notes of the analytic work that was done, within time periods ranging from one to ten years. In addition to this, for the past fifteen years, I have been able to witness, either as a therapist or as a supervisor, many other similar clinical situations. My general impression has been that these patients are quite different from one another, in terms of the seriousness of their disorders, the quality of their infantile Self, their object relations and the atmosphere that they are able to create around themselves. Indeed, they are so different that one might think they cannot belong to the same psychopathological syndrome.

Therefore, the study that will be presented in this book concerns a limited number of patients in different stages of their development, sequenced in such a way as to provide the impression of longitudinally following one single case. The point of arrival in the development of symbolic processes in the first patient marks the starting point of the second case, as the necessary premise (even if not the only one) of its evolution, and so on.

PART I

METHOD OF ENQUIRY

INTRODUCTION TO PART I

On psychoanalytic psychotherapy with patients suffering from pervasive developmental disorders

In recent years, psychotherapeutic and psychoanalytical work with children and adolescents who suffer from pervasive developmental disorders have attracted many critical and contrasting views.

In the light of aetiological considerations of a biologic and genetic character, many families, supported by associations that deal with autism, have recently launched promotional campaigns against the psychoanalytic treatment of their children in a way that I find excessive and, at times, uselessly biased. I am convinced, instead, that the therapeutic method of psychoanalysis, because of its scientific rigour and the human qualities that characterise it, has provided in the past, and will also do so in the future, a great contribution to the understanding of the autistic experience, particularly as regards the psychology of children and adolescents suffering from an arrest or a serious delay in the development of their symbolic processes.

People who attack this method often do not know it at all or know it only by hearsay, and they are very likely to think of something which no longer exists in clinical practice: its transformations in the past fifty years have been too many, and they have frequently been difficult to follow. Criticisms can also become ungenerous, when such people claim that psychoanalytic therapists might be completely uninterested in neurobiology or genetics, or that they might have no doubts at all about the therapeutic effectiveness of their work. Nothing could be further from the truth.

This is what Anne Alvarez (2004), Co-convenor with Susan Reid of the Tavistock Clinic Autism Service and Workshop, has to say about the matter:

> The question of the psychoanalytic treatment of children with autism has been surrounded by controversy. Some psychoanalysts and psychotherapists have themselves described the need for changes in technique with these children (Meltzer, 1975a; Tustin, 1981; Alvarez, 1992; Alvarez & Reid, 1999). The impairments in symbolic capacity, play, and language make an understanding of more ordinary explanatory interpretations very difficult for them. Where the autistic symptomatology is especially severe, and where not only the child's sense of existence of other people, but also his sense of self is too weak, the concepts of transference and counter-transference may seem too advanced: transference may seem to be non-existent, and a counter-transference of frustration or despair in the therapist can lead to indifference. Yet close observation may begin to reveal faint or disordered signs of relatedness which can then be amplified.
>
> The view of the Autism Workshop at the Tavistock Clinic is that, regardless of aetiology, a disorder of the capacity for social interaction may benefit from a treatment which functions via the process of social interaction itself, provided this takes account both of the nature and severity of psychopathology and the particular developmental level at which the child is functioning. The therapeutic approach is three-pronged: it addresses the child's personality, the autistic symptomatology (disorder and sometimes deviance), and the intact or spare "non-autistic" part of the child, however developmentally delayed this may be (Alvarez & Read, 1999). The psychotherapy is thus psychoanalytically, psychopathologically and developmentally informed (Alvarez, 2004, p. 96).

What is often ignored by critics is that the interpretative dimension in the psychoanalytic work with children and adolescents has deeply changed: the attempt to explain the clinical phenomena in terms of a cause-effect relationship, which in the past had led to the theory that autistic children, because of their coldness and withdrawal in their personal relationships, were simply the product of "fridge" parents, has increasingly given more space to the careful observation of their behaviours and of their communications, with the purpose of establish or rediscover shared symbolical meanings that might turn them on to psychic life. The interest in psychopathology has definitively given its place to the concern for development and the respect for "diversity".

The various symptomatologic definitions, even the most refined ones, like those linked to the recent discovery of "mirror neurones", which seems to provide firm neurological grounds to the classic descriptions of the main symptoms of autism, i.e., *the difficulty in having emotionally relevant relationships, an almost total absence of play activity and pretend play, and a delay in the development of language* (Harris, 1989), are only one part of the experience that autistic children have of themselves and of others; they only shed light on what is absent, what is missing in the children's development and their way of being and relating, compared to a model of normality, failing to grasp the complexity of what is really taking place at an "experiential" level when one is with them, close to them for so many hours, months, and years in a personal relationship that is informed only by the wish to get to know them and help them know themselves.

One immediately understands how the autistic child is much more complex than the symptomatologic definitions of autism. Behind behaviour of apparently total isolation, profoundly different experiences can be observed: moments when the child is clearly distant from us, moments when the child is against us, or with us. The problem is to decide which is the best condition to get access to such experiential moments through observation, respecting their diversity. In this sense I believe that child psychoanalysis has the responsibility to find a language that truly describes what can be observed within a therapeutic relationship with an autistic child, respecting his complexity. Indeed, there is a big difference between saying that the triad of autism is due to the inability to simulate the mental states of the other person, and claiming that it is the expression of the subject's inability to have dream thoughts about his life experience.

Simulating is not the same as dreaming, trying to imagine what the other person thinks or feels. Moreover, dreaming is not only an expression of the Self of an individual, but also of his internal objects; as Sandro Veronesi writes in his novel *XY*: "[…] the extra-sensorial perception of psychic contents […] does not mean seeing into other people's thoughts as if they were a film […] but only tuning in to them, as it were, welcoming them into oneself and being inspired by them" (Veronesi, 2010, p. 83).

CHAPTER ONE

The mind model of child psychoanalysis in clinical work with children

In this chapter I would like to talk about my psychotherapeutic work with children in general, in order to clarify, as much as possible, what is the therapeutic method of psychoanalysis and what are its main purposes. My hope is that this may facilitate and make it more interesting to read the clinical stories of some of my patients who suffered from pervasive developmental disorder, which can be found in the second and third part of this book. I will clarify this issue in the second chapter with the help of the written notes from a consultation with Carlotta, a five-year-old girl with a few phobic symptoms.

I would like to start with a question: *What are the unconscious aspects of the infantile mind that the psychoanalytic method makes accessible to a scientific exploration?*

It is well known that the work of a psychoanalytic psychotherapist and of a child psychoanalyst is mainly based on the careful observation of the unconscious aspects of the internal world of the child and of his most intimate emotional experiences, as they manifest themselves in the transference within the therapeutic relationship in a well-structured space-time context. In the past—I am referring to the early Freud and his *Studies on Hysteria* (1895d)—it was thought that the main purpose of therapy was for the patients to be able to re-experience or communicate, within the therapeutic relationship, the many painful derivatives of childhood, of a mainly sexual nature (seductions, threats of castration), which in the course of the development had been repressed since they were intolerable or unacceptable. These experiences, in their repressed state, were the basis of the inhibitions, perversions, neuroses, and peculiarities of character of the patients themselves; thus, the main purpose of the analytic work was to reconstruct their traumatic past and bring it back to light, so that the related negative affects could be explored in a situation of safety and trust. It was thought that this reconstructive work ought to be done by the analyst with a neutral attitude, without any moral judgement.

Later, after his studies on narcissism, on mourning and melancholia, on falling in love and reactions to physical illness, Freud (1923b, pp. 3–59) formulated his structural theory of the mind in *The Ego and the Id*, introducing the famous image of the Ego as the servant of two masters: the instinctual part of the personality, i.e., the Id, and a powerful and destructive unconscious morality, i.e., the Superego. The past was still important, no longer as a reserve of traumatic memories but as an expression of an unconscious, phylogenetic, and ontogenetic, heritage in which contradictory impulses of life and death, love and hate were in a state of mutual, constant struggle.

The task of the analyst, therefore, was to try to recognise this state of things and attempt to modify the pathological defences erected by the Ego in the course of the patient's infantile development in order to cope with the destructive impulses coming from the Id and the sadistic aspects of the Superego, replacing them with other defences, more suitable to reality, thus allowing adult sexuality and love to emerge. In this situation, the analyst kept a neutral, detached attitude, but at the same time he was aware of the "evil" nature of Man, trying to be patient and tolerant towards the thoughts and behaviours of his patients, who often showed their resistance against letting go of their neuroses.

Until then, it was thought that children could not be analysed as patients following the psychoanalytic method, and the clinical case of Little Hans shows evidence of this. Indeed, Freud wrote this essay as a complement of his studies on the sexual theory and not as a clinical example of child analysis. He claimed that children, for a number of reasons, were not suitable to the type of psychological therapy that he had "discovered".

Therefore, child psychoanalysis did not originate with Freud. Its birth, instead, is linked to the clinical work of three great women: Hermine von Hug-Hellmuth (1871–1924), Melanie Klein (1882–1960), and Anna Freud (1895–1982), who in the 1920s, 1930s, and 1940s respectively, in different contexts and with different theoretical premises, gave great impulse to the psychoanalytic studies of children. Other valid contributions came after World War II, with the baby and young child observation studies of Esther Bick (1964) and Martha Harris (1977), which greatly contributed to the understanding of development in children and to the training of child psychotherapists at the Tavistock Clinic in London.

Psychoanalytic work with children, even very young ones, introduced radical changes in perspective within psychoanalytical thinking, particularly in those areas of experience that Freud considered as essential to know, in order to effectively fight against the neurotic symptoms of his adult patients: "[…] first their past, particularly their childhood past; second, the sexual content of the memories or phantasies connected with this past; and third, the powerful repressive forces that kept the lid on this seething pot" (Alvarez, 1992, p. 1).

In the work with children, the effort to reconstruct past experiences became secondary: in the here and now of the therapeutic interaction, the child analyst immediately had to face the task of "tuning in" to the forces that promoted development, rather than of understanding the forces against it. Therapy became a process of knowledge more oriented to the future than to the past. Moreover, it began to be noticed that, in their play, children showed interest in their parents, particularly in the body and the mind of the mother, from the very first days of post-natal life, and that on that primary relational experience they built their own view of the world, imbued with values, anxieties, worries, and phantasies that could not simply be related to sexuality or to the traumatic effects of reality. Finally, evidence was gathered that in the economy and development of psychic life, the Superego, by now called "internal objects", performed important functions of containment, protection, and guidance, and it was thus the basis for the child's stability and mental growth, and not simply a psychic instance at the service of repression. The reconstructive work of the past, therefore, left the field free to the discovery of those processes that were the roots of the emotional and mental development of children, which manifested themselves within the analytic relationship.

There was an increased awareness that what the child transferred in the here and now of the therapeutic experience was no longer the repressed part of a past that had to be reconstructed, but "mental states" in search of a container-mind able to think and give meaning to them.

The discovery that the child, from a very early age, had a very complex "psychic reality", in a state of constantly oscillating relationship with the external world by means of complex projective and introjective processes, showed the need, on the part of the psychoanalytic therapist, not to obliterate the mental and emotional experiences born in him as a consequence of his participation to the therapeutic experience and the encounter with the internal world of the child: the so-called countertransference.

The quality of the countertransference response became—together with the playroom—a fundamental feature for the promotion of the externalisation and exploration of internal object relations in the case of less seriously ill children and of the communication of very primitive mental states through projective identification in the case of more seriously ill children. The therapeutic method of child psychoanalysis brought forward the idea that the birth and the growth of the personality of a child—particularly regarding the processes of individuation and separation, and the development of symbolic processes and verbal language—were closely linked to the realisation and the overcoming, within the therapeutic relationship, of specific transference configurations and their evolution, through interpretative work, into stable mental structures as a foundation for the capacity to think (Meltzer, 1967; Joseph, 1989; Houzel, 2004). Quoting Meltzer, we could then say, at the end of this brief historical digression:

> [...] the therapeutic method of psychoanalysis is based on the patient's capacity to experience a transference relationship, and to tolerate if not actively to participate in his analyst's description and investigation of this transference relationship. The therapeutic benefit for the patient is found in the evolution of the transference, an evolution that depends above all on the meeting of the transference with a congruent counter-transference, which the patient can recognize and use towards a goal of comprehension rather than action (Meltzer, 1986a, in: *Sincerity and other Works*, 1994, p. 552).

Nowadays we are able, in the course of the therapeutic process, to recognise different configurations of the transference, and to link them to various forms of psychopathology that we encounter in children and adolescents, such as two-dimensionality and post-autistic immaturity, confusional infantile and adolescent psychoses, borderline states and infantile neuroses with great benefits regarding the differentiation and modulation of the therapeutic intervention.

The spectrum of these clinical situations can bluntly be enclosed within these two polarities in which, on one hand, we observe children who are "almost incapable of developing a transference situation", who are emotionally still unable to live in the world and in their bodies as a "life space" and have a very primitive relationship with time; and on the other, we see children whose unconscious fantasy and subjective experience of time have structurally evolved, thus enabling them to develop a transference with their analyst, but who are still immature because they are unable to face the difficulties of separation and separateness, oedipal pain and the loss of their grandiose infantile identity.

Finally, I would like to point out how the discoveries of child analysis, both Kleinian and post-Kleinian—and particularly Klein's concept of "psychic reality"—have contributed to the modification of the entrenched idea that infantile development follows a linear and consequential progression in stages, introducing a developmental concept that simple chronology cannot explain. They have shown how in the child's personality, temperament, and character feature there are very specific and individual factors (psychic reality is an individual construction) that can influence, positively or negatively, every single phase or developmental stage, determining the modalities of transition between one stage and the next, the appreciation or rejection of a single developmental phase.

Studying the transference, the child psychotherapist will then have to shed light on those characteristics of the psychic reality of the child that can influence his development, positively or negatively, to clarify the relationships between "mental states" and developmental stages (Waddell, 1998) and thus to differentiate what is pathological from what is primitive in object relations, and regressive aspects from defensive ones in narcissism.

CHAPTER TWO

An example of psychoanalytic consultation with children: the clinical case of Carlotta (C)

At this point I would like to illustrate what I said earlier with the help of the notes of the first consultation session with C, a five-year-old girl. My purpose in discussing this piece of clinical work here is to show how a particular receptive and listening attitude adopted by an experienced, sensitive adult, in the context of a setting that is well structured and sufficiently free from external interferences, allows, in just a few sequences, the child to reveal some deep aspects of her relations and emotional life. This, in turn, facilitates the therapist's understanding, and my own as a supervisor, of the main characteristics of the little girl's personality structure so to formulate a few interpretative hypotheses about her symptoms, which will be investigated later in the following sessions and finally shared with her parents.

C is a five-year-old girl attending a private nursery. She has a sister who is two years her senior. Her parents want a consultation because for a few months, before going to kindergarten, C has started vomiting (despite having an empty stomach, since she never eats her breakfast), or panicking as a consequence of a simple reprimand, saying that she has heartache and that she cannot breathe. C never shows her anger or rebellion, and she often shows—both at home and at the kindergarten—an excessively complacent attitude, despite being often in the grip of feelings of anxiety when faced with something that was not programmed by her, or anything unpredictable.

First Observation session

> C arrives with both parents, and they all come in; she is holding on to her mother, but she smiles at me and looks at me with curiosity. She is a beautiful, thriving child (which I did not expect her to be), with a lively, curious gaze, staring at me. I introduce myself, and her mother makes her notice that it is as she had said to her that I am a doctor without a white coat! She invites her to ask me the thing that mattered to her. C remains silent, and her mother says that she wanted to know if I am a kind of doctor that gives children injections. I say that I do not, I am not a doctor like the one she knows, I deal with the things that make children worried, and I wanted to know her because mummy and daddy told me that there is something that worries her, a lot. I know that she sometimes feels bad here (I point at her stomach) and then she feels like vomiting, and this is certainly not nice at all … C nods and looks at me. I add that in order to understand what makes her feel bad we will have to get to know each other, and the best way to do that is to play together for a while. We still do not know each other, and she must find all this a bit strange, maybe she is a little worried, and also curious … C nods. I show her the toy box and I explain to her what we will do together.
>
> Once I conclude my brief speech I tell her that perhaps she now wants to see what's inside; I ask her if she prefers to play on the table or on the carpet, and she chooses the latter.
>
> She begins with the plasticine and asks me what it is. She gives me a bit of white plasticine to warm it up, telling me that also her teachers in the kindergarten warm it up for the children. I remark that she has found something that she knows here, where everything is so new …
>
> After that, she gets interested in the little dolls representing the various family members. She looks at them one by one very attentively. At this point I ask her if her parents can wait for her outside. She willingly accepts it.
>
> She notices that a stocking that the grandmother is knitting is incomplete and wants to know who has knitted it. She is fascinated by it, mainly by the knitting needles, and she handles them for a while. She asks me their name. When I tell her that they are called "*ferri*" (knitting needles are called in Italian "*ferri*" which means "made with iron") she replies immediately that they are made of wood, not of iron; smiling, I tell her that she is right. She looks at the other members of the family, attributing a role to

each of them: grandparents, mother, father (she uses the "older brother" character, but they are similar in height), the older daughter, the baby (it is swaddled, and initially she does not understand what sex it is); the "father" character becomes the uncle. She notices that the older sister is wearing her pyjamas (a dress, in fact). C tells me that her aunt is pregnant, has a baby in her belly, adding that she found out about it just the other day (in our initial interview, her parents told me that the news has been circulating for quite some time, and that C often strokes her aunt's belly, saying "hello" to her little cousin). I tell her that she must have been taken by surprise by it but she replies that she was not, she already knew about it. C adds that when her aunt noticed that her belly had grown, she thought that she had eaten too much, while C herself already knew that it was a baby instead!

Commentary

I would like to point out a few things that stand out in these initial moments of the encounter between the child and the therapist. First of all we see how the child tries to "size up" the therapist, when a person that she does not know comes into her life; with the help of her mother the girl tries to understand whether this person is benevolent or dangerous. She fears that the therapist might be like the doctor at the A&E unit, where she was taken recently because of an accident to her arm. The therapist is immediately aware of the narrow gap between trust and fear in the child's expectations when she meets her for the first time. The child compares the mother to the therapist, and when she discovers that there are no major disharmonies or inconsistencies between them about the meaning of what is happening, she is reassured and makes herself available to the exploration of the new relationship and the new place without her parents. One can then observe an interesting second phenomenon linked to the fact that the little girl begins to take an interest in the contents of the toy-box and the play material that "the doctor" has prepared for her: first the plasticine, then the family characters. The child, driven by her curiosity, finds things, recognises functions, roles, and conditions that she already knows. She is clearly intelligent and curious, even if rather controlled in her emotional expressions and her play activity. She would simply like to have a chat with the doctor and talk to her about the multitude of people, things and activities that fill her life, but she cannot hide her emotions and her worries completely. She notices that the plasticine is hard and that the hands of an adult are needed to warm it up. But perhaps she also wants to say that it is not always pleasant to be at the kindergarten, because one feels small and dependent there. She is interested in the grandma character, who is knitting, and she seems to be keen on knitting, but perhaps she also realises that some of her curiosities cannot be easily fulfilled, and that there are things that are not easy to understand; she sees the sister character wearing a dress, and she thinks that she is wearing a strange kind of pyjamas, as is she wanted to draw attention on the topic of darkness, or on the experience of going to bed. Finally, the baby character also draws her attention, making her feel so anxious as to trigger a little manic reaction, when she claims—by making reference to her aunt—that she knows everything about how mummies get their bellies big. "It is clear that they don't get it big because they eat too much", she says, showing that her certainties lose their solidity the moment when she explores her infantile body. In a very short time span we see a child that talks about her life; but in doing so she also shows us the most hidden emotions and curiosities that characterise her thoughts and feelings about her experiences of dependence and autonomy at the kindergarten (perhaps with some persecutory moments), her curiosity about babies and female creativity (with some jealousy and envy), her fascination with an object—the grandma doll—that seems to represent the mystery of a thinking mind, wrapped in itself, that can create objects that are precious because they are custom made, specially crafted, and who represents another idea of femininity, of a mother. The child is already unconsciously providing her therapist with the agenda for their next meetings.

> [...] C then looks at the bag containing the farm animals; she takes it and I offer my help to open it, but she says that she can manage by herself. First of all, she looks at the pieces of the fence and puts them together; she forgets one of them in the heap of the animals; the paw of one of those that she uses is twisted, but she does not care. Then she takes the animals and groups them in families, putting them into the enclosure. One of the horses cannot stand on its legs, so I help her by spreading its legs a bit; she manages to make another horse stand by herself. This first enclosure is small, but curiously she leaves out one of the pieces, despite having seen it.
>
> She moves the enclosure next to the box, so the two animals with twisted paws can manage to stand. She also rests the horses against the box. Then she puts together the "cow family", noticing that the "mummy" is the "swollen one". At first I think she is talking about its belly, but then she

clarifies that she is full of milk. There a few gaps in the enclosure, and the animals want to run away; the dog is watching over one of the gaps.

Something makes a little noise. I do not remember what it is. She remarks: "It makes a 'cri cri' sound, like when I eat, I am a little mouse, I eat cheese!" She makes sweet nibbling sounds. I ask her what she likes, and she replies: "I like salami with bread and cheese! Mmm!" I then ask her what she does not like at all: "I don't like milk, it has that funny smell, you know? And its taste, when you drink it, you know?"

The grandmother goes to check the animals, so that they do not run away. Grandpa says to grandma that he went to school, where the headmaster reprimanded him because of his scruffy clothes. Putting myself in grandma's shoes, I repeat the words of grandpa, as if to say, "Did I hear that right?" Carlotta repeats the words, laughing, without adding anything else.

She takes away the animals to put in some new ones. This time it is the geese (mother, older sister with the younger brothers behind), then the sheep, and finally the hedgehog, the otter, and the rabbit (these animals are bigger than the others). I tell her that there is also the little mouse lying abandoned among the others, because I think she might not have noticed it, but she does not consider it. She then takes the bag with the dinosaurs, asking me to help her open it (it is closed like the one with the farm animals, which she had earlier been able to open by herself). I notice that one needs some help to let the dinosaurs go free ... C looks at them, makes them bite things, and she remarks that two kinds of stegosaurus of different sizes are in fact a mother and her son. She takes the crocodile and lets it bite her finger; fascinated, she notices that its mouth is stained with blood, and then she adds that we all have a mouth stained with blood, because it is red, the colour of blood, and so are our tongues. She tries to stick her finger into the mouth of a small tyrannosaurus, noticing that her finger does not get inside completely, whereas if it were long enough it would get all the way into the belly of the crocodile.

Commentary

If in the first part of the session the child talks about the people in her life, in the second part she highlights some aspects of her infantile self, and her worries and anxieties mainly concern the relationships between part objects: mouth/teeth—mouth/breast—nipple/tongue.

C plays with the animals; first she opens the bag with the farm animals, and then the one with the wild animals, among which there are some prehistoric ones, like dinosaurs. The therapist is immediately aware that the child asks for help only for the second bag, despite the bags have the same kind of seal. She makes her notice this, jokingly, in the attempt to make her stop and think about why she cannot open it by herself. Is she tired or particularly frightened by the wild, prehistoric animals? Or is she anxious because she knows how to manage the farm animals and knows their habits and needs, but she does not what to do with the wild ones, where to place and to control them, and for this reason she finds them unreliable, unpredictable, violent and undecipherable?

As a matter of fact, even when she plays with the farm animals there is something that she cannot control. She is very good at grouping them into families or types; however, the enclosure is not sufficient for all of them: there is only space for one family at a time, so she starts putting the horse family in first, then she takes them out and replaces them with the cow family (with mummy cow and her udders full of milk); then she moves on to the geese, then the sheep and finally the "big" animals (including a little mouse), which are not really a family in a biological sense. The surprising thing is that these animals want to run away from this enclosure, and therefore she must employ dogs (or grandma) to guard the holes. Grandma is now back on the scene, but this time she is no longer a good seamstress/knitter, but a capable farmer who can look after her animals, as well as a wife who is not very mindful of Grandpa's clothes: he complains to her about the criticism from the head teacher for his scruffy clothes. Finally, the character of the mouse appears which the child introduces on stage in what the therapist considers a significantly emotional manner. While the cow full of milk is in the enclosure, the child steps on an object that lets out a little squeak. The child (maybe afraid of having done something wrong) immediately associates the squeak to the sound of the teeth of a mouse gnawing on a piece of cheese. "I"—says C—"am the little mouse eating the cheese", quickly adding that she finds the milk of mummy cow disgusting, because it stinks and tastes bad; she prefers other types of food. The interesting thing is that after this sequence C is unable to see the toy mouse lying abandoned among the other animals outside the enclosure. The therapist invites her to play with the toy mouse, but the child ignores her suggestion.

The play activity of the child with the wild animals introduces more primitive themes that have to do with biting mouths full of blood, long fingers entering into mouths, pushing hard as deeply as possible, into the stomach and the belly. The child seems to be talking about two types of violence: biting and being penetrated. Unfortunately, since the beginning of the session the therapist has been absorbed in the task of warming up the piece of plasticine, and she does not follow the child's train of thought. One wonders what would have happened if the therapist had asked the child to talk to her about her eating difficulties, her refusal to have breakfast, and about the vomiting fits that she had recently had, before going to school; or if she had showed the child a possible link between the disgusting milk coming from the cow's udders and the red mouths of the wild animals. One cannot say, and maybe it is useless to wonder about that. However, one should not fail to notice the "gravity" and the "seriousness" of what the child tells us through her play activity; intuitively, we they may be ascribed to her confused feelings about the goodness not only of mother's milk, but also of the way in which it was given to her, or the way in which the nipple was put into her mouth to feed her; and also about the goodness of her own "mouse-like" mouth and teeth, which are perhaps crocodile teeth (a kind of confusion which is the basis of most eating disorders in early infancy).

> I am still handling my piece of plasticine making a long and thin roll with it; she sees it and takes it, then she ties into a knot and shows it to me. She folds it in half, horizontally joining its two ends, then she folds it again vertically, creating a compact shape that makes me think of something folded onto itself, and I talk to her about it. I tell her that our time is up; she looks disappointed but does not protest. I notice that she is sorry, but I say that we can meet again next Tuesday. She looks excited and repeats emphatically "Yes, yes!" Her attitude is a bit contrived, but in a happy way, which is quite typical of children. As she leaves, C tells her parents that she wants to come back, and they look relieved. We fix an appointment for the following week.

Commentary

We can see that the session ends in a minor key. As the final goodbye approaches, the child seems to emotionally distance herself from the relationship with the doctor and to find shelter in omnipotent control and (defensive) insincerity. I would not be so sure that the child might come back for her next session so easily, as she seems to make everyone think at this point. I ask myself whether she will vomit on her way to the doctor, as she does before getting to school. Let us see why. The child's doubts about the goodness of the milk and the nipple seem to extend to the doctor who has prepared a plasticine sausage roll for her. For a moment, C lets herself be involved with this object, and she ties it as if it were a woollen thread. Then she shows it to the doctor (the knot makes one think of those used by the grandma doll when she knits), as if expecting a compliment from her, or as an invitation to do something together, to play together, which is what her maternal grandmother maybe used to do with her (we know that until the age of three, when C started going to the kindergarten, she was with her grandmother every time her mother had to go somewhere, even if, more recently, the child has refused to leave her home and go to grandma's house). This moment of contact does not last long: the child immediately withdraws in herself, entering into a mental state that is not easy to decipher. She starts to fold the plasticine roll repeatedly, making it more compact; the knot disappears within a shapeless lump. What did the child feel about the doctor when she showed her the knot and did not feel appreciated for what she did? Did she have doubts about her goodness? Is she thinking about doing something with the plasticine all by herself? Whom did she identify with when she withdraws into her "shell", disappointed by the end of the session, without the time or chance to play together? Does she perhaps want the therapist to feel what one feels when the knot of an affective link is cut, or when one's expectations are not met? What happens when one misses a stitch while knitting? The wish to play with the doctor, or the wish to be on her own come and go at the same pace of the sun appearing or disappearing among the clouds on a day in spring.

How do we know what a child feels and thinks?

At this point of the discussion, after listening to the clinical material of C we can finally pause to think about how we know what the child feels and thinks in her unconscious, as well as about the nature of the conclusions that we intend to share with her and with her parents at the end of the consultation. It is commonly believed that we can understand the emotional experience of a child or an adolescent simply by putting ourselves in her shoes and imagining what we might feel or think if we were in her position, her mind and her body. We think we know a child by identifying with her, projecting on her, or into her, emotions and thoughts, which belong to our own mental and emotional personal experience. Sometimes we can even put all of ourselves into her.

The empathetic attitude of the therapist is based on the conviction that the child and we are very similar in many human motivations, attitudes, and basic emotional reactions. If the child tells us that the teacher is "bad", we try to understand her anger imagining how we would have felt in her position; we try to envisage the "badness" of the teacher on the basis of similar personal experiences. However, we also know by experience that empathy is a rather blunt guide in our understanding of a child, and that there are many things that can deceive us and lead us to draw wrong conclusions about her way of feeling and facing things, especially when we are not able to grasp her diversity and we assume that she is altogether similar to us in our way of feeling and thinking. In doing this, we run the risk of seeing too many things about ourselves in the child. How many times have we heard a parent tell us "my child is exactly as I was when I was a child" and we have grasped this statement as an attempt to deny the diversities of the child? What choices do we have then? C's doctor shows us that there is another possibility, which lies in an *attitude* that we might call *receptive*. Unlike empathy, when we use our mind to get into the mind of a child, a receptive attitude implies taking the child inside ourselves as she is, with what she feels and thinks in that moment, using our mind as an instrument that is sensitive to the vibrations and the echo of her projections. In this way we think we know her through what she makes us feel about herself through her projections and her communications, which are often nonverbal, or through what she makes us become, all the people whom she identifies us with. The receptivity I am talking about must not be confused with passivity; on the contrary, it is a process by which we let ourselves be involved and taken in by the projections and the identifications of the child without being overwhelmed by the emotional reactions that these arouse in us. This implies, on our part, an active and continuous act of listening to what she makes us feel at an intimate level. It is a form of passionate knowledge, in which feelings help us support understanding more than acting.

In psychoanalytic language we might say that we know the child through what she deposits in our mind when she transforms us into transference objects (Freud) or receptacles (the notion of toilet breast of Donald Meltzer) of her most primitive or painful projections, either verbal or non-verbal, through projective identification (Melanie Klein).

How do we draw a map of the internal world of a child?

So far, I have tried to illustrate different ways with which we observe children, in the attempt to draw a truthful "map" of their internal and external object relations. With the help of C's clinical material, we can now try to learn more about the features of this "map" and to understand how it can be drawn in order for it to be understandable both for the child and her parents.

At a quick glance, C seems a child fit for her age from an emotional and intellectual point of view. She can let her parents help her win the fears and the resistance that she feels about the new experience of a consultation, but she is also able to let them leave the play room without making too much fuss when the doctor asks her to do so. We can see how she is well disposed about the room; she freely chooses where to sit, she opens the toy box by herself without difficulty or inhibitions and is available to acknowledge her need for dependence. We also notice how quickly she borrows helpful pointers from other situations in life in order to make sense of her new relationship with the doctor. She seems to be saying to herself: "If things here are not like at the A&E, then they are like at the kindergarten; if here the doctor does not give me an injection, then she must be like my teacher, who warms up the plasticine when it is hard." Moreover, through the use of verbal language, the child shows an adequate symbolic development and a good awareness of herself, her own personal boundaries and of those of other people. She is curious, sometimes in a sincere and enthusiastic manner, whereas other times she uses her curiosity to criticise, to keep everything under control and to be a little braggart. On the whole, she is a beautiful, intelligent, clever girl who shows that she has reached a good differentiation, in terms of her personality development, between her Self and her Objects and that she has acknowledged the fact that her personal world and the world of the people who are close to her are realities that are full of emotions, thoughts, interests and expectations which can all be shared.

So far so good, then!

However, C's parents tell us that there is a "lump" of reactions, feelings and emotions in the child's experience which prevents her from managing the anxiety and the confusion that she may experience in situations related to her developmental stage, such as being reprimanded, leaving her home to go to the kindergarten and dealing with her aunt's pregnancy. Are these parents wrong to be so worried about their child? How can we consider her anxious crises, her vomiting and the trouble with her "belly"? Once again, it is the child herself who helps us. As you read in my comments and in the clinical material, there are many interesting things that she tells us, through her behaviour, her play activity with the toys, her verbal and non-verbal communications regarding herself and her life, regarding her curiosities and her emotions, which can help us draw our "map": the generally controlling and rather complacent attitude towards the consultation and the therapist; the slight anxiety that she experiences inside and outside the consultation room, every time she is faced with something that makes her feel small, ignorant, and needy (the bag with the fears and prehistoric animals that does not open, her pregnant aunt, her sister in pyjamas, the hard plasticine at the kindergarten, the enclosure that does not hold); the intensity of her curiosity for the knitting of the grandma character and the positive and negative feelings about her activity and her functions as a mother and a wife; the comment on the "badness" of the cow milk; the moment she is identified with the hungry little mouse; the game in which she sticks her finger into the mouths of the wild and prehistoric animals reaching their belly-tail; and finally, the way in which she ties and unties a knot, at the end of the session, using the plasticine roll prepared by her doctor.

In the light of this material, I am inclined to think that C is telling us two parallel stories: with the first story, she wants to tell us something about her phantasies, feelings, and anxieties about night-time or absent parents. The main features of her "script" are the big belly of the aunt character, the swollen udders of the mother cow, the enclosures that do not hold, from which animals can escape, the watch dog, the hungry, neglected and squeaking little mouse, the mouths full of blood of the dinosaurs and the finger stuck into the belly of the prehistoric animals. C seems to be telling us: "When I go to bed at night or when I have to go to the kindergarten, I feel hungry and neglected. I know that, somewhere, there is a breast-mother full of milk and a belly-shelter-mother, but I am told that she is no longer mine like in the past, because now she is gone back to her old owner, daddy, who might in the future (just like uncle) lend her to a baby brother of mine. I also understand that mother doesn't dislike all this at all, and that she finds it pleasant to do certain things with daddy that fill her breast with milk and make her belly swell just like my aunt. I am often upset by this situation and I have the worst thoughts: I am afraid that daddy might fill mummy up with bad things that make her dirty or violent, or that he might hurt her, devour her, and bite her. I am not sure about this either. Sometimes I think that I would like to be a grown-up like mummy, have her beautiful body and take her place next to daddy. However, I realise that it's not easy to escape from my room, even if it would only take a little hole to leave my den, just like the little mouse. I would like to hide in mummy and daddy's bedroom or get into their big bed, but they forbid me to do it. In all this story, there is something I don't understand and that particularly upsets me, because I don't know how all this can happen to me; sometimes I feel so starved and neglected that I would like to eat my mummy up or to enter into her with some force. Then, I am afraid to damage and lose her, so I never want to let her go during the day, or I am afraid to make my daddy so angry that he becomes as dangerous as grandma's barking watch dog when he chases away the thieves (including the little mice) from the enclosures. I feel so bad that I think that he might send me away and never let me come back home again."

The second story is about her daytime parents, with characters like the grandmother who knits and puts her animals to sleep; the grandfather who seems to have an important social role; the farm animals; a country lifestyle, with people cooking, making clothes, and knitting. The grandparents are two parents that are perhaps a bit too old to make love, towards whom the child seems to have more positive feelings, because they make her feel "big" and make her take part in their life, unlike the night-time parents, who cut her off from their intimacy, which she cannot see as good. These two stories make us think that there might be two children: the daytime girl and the night-time girl, who seem to be not very integrated; they do not talk much to each other and, at times, the fantasies and anxieties of the night-time girl manage to invade the emotional experiences of the daytime girl.

CHAPTER THREE

The eyes and the mind (1): on the observational processes in clinical work with children

In this chapter I would like to develop a few very personal ideas on the relationship between the eyes and the mind in psychoanalytic psychotherapeutic work with children and adolescents. To do so, I will make use of material from different sources: clinical material from the initial assessment meetings with a seven-year-old boy, not particularly ill and therefore quite ready to get to know his emotions and his deepest thoughts; and from a psychotherapy session with a young adolescent, with Asperger's syndrome, who was still stuck on his beliefs and unable to enter into a world of shared meanings. My two clinical cases will be preceded by observational material from one of my colleagues, which she gathered within the ward of neonatal intensive therapy where she worked; and literary material from *The Blue Bear* (2002), a novel by the American writer Lynn Schooler, which clearly illustrates the impact of artistic creation on symbolic development. Finally, I will discuss two poems by Tagore, one on the birth and the other on the death of a child, to exemplify how a poet can observe and give shape to certain fundamental human experiences.

In the previous chapter we have seen that as child psychoanalysts we are constantly involved in the detailed observation of the behaviour of our young patients. It is a careful direct, non-intrusive observation which takes place within a very precise setting: very regular, safe, simple, and sufficiently intimate, and, unlike other observational modalities, does not avail itself of any technical aid, like the video-recording and microanalysis of the image, or of the support of notes taken directly during the sessions. It is an observation which is often followed, at the end of every session, by the detailed annotation of the sequences that have been observed, and by a discussion of our written notes within individual or group supervisions. Apparently, we try to do what a mother does, day by day, with her baby, or what an educator does when she tries to understand the children she has been entrusted with. I say "apparently", because, in fact, the purpose of our observations within the analytic setting is quite different from that of a mother in the family, or that of an educator in an educational context. We do not want to educate the child; our sole purpose is to get to know his internal world and to help him to know himself.

But what is the link between observing the child and understanding what is inside him?

In a reflection on gestalt themes, Wittgenstein (1953) stated that there is no "immaculate", neutral and purely passive perception, and that the relationship between a thing and its image is not analogous to the one between an original and a copy. In perception there is "a thought that is echoed in seeing" (Bodei, 2008, p. 19).

What is echoed, then, when a child psychoanalyst listens to, and looks at a child, determinedly trying to understand the emotional life of his young patients? What is the thought that is echoed in his observing and listening to a child within the analytic situation, and how is it that this thought engages the child and activates or accelerates the development of his mental life?

The answer is: our countertransference, that is, those emotions, feelings, conscious or unconscious states of mind that are aroused in us by the direct participation in the infantile transference of our patients, with whom we use our analytic skills for understanding. Psychoanalytic observation is not, therefore, an "objective" observation, in the traditional sense of the term, in which the subjective and emotional variables of the observing psychoanalyst are excluded as much as possible; on the contrary, the observation must favour the analyst's deep contact with his own unconscious, and with those aspects of his unconscious that are activated by the therapeutic encounter with his patient. The encounter inside the analytic room with children that are developmentally very damaged has introduced new contents in our inner experience, difficult to tolerate and to understand, sometimes disturbing, associated to long periods of impasse in the therapeutic work or to prolonged situations of great incommunicability, psychic solipsism, and impossibility to find any shared meanings. This has led to the need to improve our unconscious receptivity and capacity for deeper identification *vis-à-vis* these very primitive aspects of the patients' mental functioning, radically modifying our observational stance within the therapy room.

Once again, I found my bearings and I made sense of this change in Dr Meltzer's scientific contribution. I am referring to a few studies on this topic carried out by Dr Meltzer in the early 1970s as a completion of what he wrote in *The Psychoanalytic Process* (1967), arguably his most inspired work, in which he investigated the nature of the analytic process from the point of view of the patient's unconscious, but neglected to study the impact of infantile transference on the mind of the analyst and on his countertransference.

Encouraged in his further investigative effort by Bion's work in *Attention and Interpretation* (1970), Dr Meltzer published, a few years later, two papers which appear very technical at first, but have, in fact, great epistemological depth. They describe how the analyst gets to know his patients: I am referring to "Routine and inspired interpretation: their relation to the weaning process in analysis" (1973) and "Temperature and distance as technical dimensions of interpretation" (1976).

In the first paper he assumes that the analyst's interpretative function may oscillate between two extreme situations, i.e., "routine interpretation and inspired interpretation".

> I am going to employ a polarizing concept for investigating the range of analytic interpretative activity by assuming two extreme types: in one of these the analyst listens and observes the behaviour of the patient which comes to assume a pattern or gestalt in his mind, to which he then applies certain aspects of his theoretical equipment in an explanatory way, while in the latter, the analyst, exposed to the activities of the patient, has an experience that is essentially personal, which he then uses, with the aid of his theoretical equipment, to explore the meaning of the relationship going on at the moment in his room (Meltzer, 1973, p. 292).

In his second paper, Dr Meltzer once again deals with these two polarities of the analyst's interpretative function, this time from the point of view of the *"ingenuity of verbal expression"* (Meltzer, 1976, p. 375). He differentiates between a more "committed" language, used in order to make meta-psychological statements (interpretation proper) and an uncertain, "meditative" language, used in order to express exploratory thinking (interpretative activity). He describes two dimensions of inventive verbal activity in "meditative" language, i.e., temperature and distance, which he considers of fundamental importance to remain in touch with the most profound and primitive mental states of the patients' emotional life. Originally, both from a historical and a developmental perspective, they seem to have a rhythmical and tonal representation, and that only later find a verbal expression through the poetic function of the metaphor, of myths and dreams, where the internal world is revealed through the shapes of the external world and the vocabulary that the child has already built in order to accumulate and communicate information about the external world.

These two polarities in the interpretative function, as described by Dr Meltzer, show how in the analyst's eyes—in his observational function and attitude—two types of thought and language are echoed. In the first one, the act of seeing is supported and guided by well-tested knowledge, based on facts and theories that are already known, by classic interpretative "scientific" language and by an easily recognisable countertransference experience. In the second polarity, the act of seeing is supported and guided by a more intuitive knowledge, as mysterious in its origin and its meaning as a dream, by a more poetic language, metaphorical, full of paradoxes and musical accents, and by emotions which are not easily decipherable in their meaning.

These different ways of looking characterise different mental experiences and express different qualities of attention: the former is more similar to a waking state, where the Ego of the individual is busy removing, choosing and concentrating, while the latter is more similar to a resting/sleeping, dreaming state, imaginatively conjecturing, and freely associating, in which the Ego stops wanting, detaches itself from life, does not pose practical problems, indeed becomes "less tense, but more extended" (Bergson, 1919).

Towards the end of his life, Dr Meltzer often stated that the psychoanalytical method is an observational method, and he described the observer's state as a mainly restful but also extremely vigilant state, and he compared it to "waiting in the dark for deer, grazing at night, seen by their flashing tails [...]" (Williams, 2005).

At this point, as I promised in my premise, I would like to examine a few situations, which have helped me acknowledge the meaning and the importance of these "sudden flashes", of these "dream thoughts" for the mental and emotional development of a child, or of the most primitive parts of the personality of an individual. I would like to show you what happens when this creative union/alliance between the eyes and the mind does not take place, as in "autistic thought", and, in contrast with that, how it can find its best expression in the language of poetry. Through the examples I am presenting you will be able to notice the constant presence of two characters, whose ways of observing and interpreting reality reflect the two polarities described by Dr Meltzer.

Holding on to the dream

First of all I would like to invite you to read a story I found in a modern novel, called *The Blue Bear*:

> [...] I had first met Michio Hoshino only a month before, when he had telephoned out of the blue and asked to charter me for a month to work on a film for a Tokyo-based broadcasting company. Now we were in Glacier Bay National Park, a few days from the end of five-week trip. We'd stopped off in this small cove to document a phenomenon left behind by the retreat of the Ice Age ... All around us stumps and tree trunks the colour of driftwood protruded from a surface of loose till.
>
> [...]
>
> Some of the interstadial wood has been carbon-dated at seven thousand years' I explained.
>
> [...]
>
> Michio probed ahead with his folded tripod, using it as a staff to stabilize his footing, then stopped beside a stump and braced his hand against it before swinging his heavy pack to the ground. "Please say again how this happened?" he asked, unfolding the legs of the tripod and working it level into the ground.
>
> [...]

"Well, during the last ice age, the glaciers advanced very rapidly," I said, sweeping a hand before my chest to indicate the flow of the ice coming down from the head of Muir Inlet below us. "And a tremendous amount of water was flowing along the sides, washing all this gravel and sand down from back in the valleys. The outflow just buried the forest alive. The gravel covered I this deep"—here I pointed to the top of the splintered stump, level with my head—"and the ice rode forward on the new surface, shearing off the trees as it went".

Michio dug a camera body from his pack and snapped it onto the tripod. "And when the glacier started to melt, water washed everything away?"

I nodded, then shrugged out of my pack. "Right. Washed all the sand and gravel down the fjord and left the forest behind. It's not petrified, just preserved for thousands of yeas by a lack of oxygen during the time it was buried".

Michio looked thoughtful for a moment, then stroked the platinum smooth face of the stamp. "Seven thousand years". He sighed. "It makes life seem so short".

[...]

He adjusted the camera while we talked, dusted the lens with a small brush, made a minute adjustment of the focus, and attached a shutter cord. "So," he finally said. "The forest is like a bear, going unto sleep in the winter and coming up again". I nodded in agreement and arched my spine to let the breeze cool the skin beneath my pack.

[...]

There was something I wanted to ask him, a favour I'd been chewing on for days,

[...]

I motioned to his camera, trying to sound casual. "Would you teach me a little something about photography?"

Michio didn't reply as he snapped the picture and rewound the camera, then glanced at the lowering sun and clicked the shutter again.

[...]

Michio squinted into the viewfinder a few moments more, nodded, and the stepped back, motioning toward the camera: "Dozo. Please do you want to see?"

> Giddily, I bent down to the camera and put my eye to the viewfinder, I pulled back—amazed—and looked at the stump, then lowered my head again to the camera. What I saw in the camera was not like anything I had seen with my eyes. The stump, framed to pass from the top of the picture, formed a perfect balance with a composition of varicoloured stones jumbled at its base. The sweeping lines of the roots drew my eye along the grain of the ancient tree to the edge of the frame and seemed to suggest that something outside the picture—perhaps the soul of the tree—was standing and looking down on the perfect waiting stillness of the stones cradled in the curve of its roots like an infant in the arms of its mother. Where I had seen only a random arrangement of rocks and deadwood, Michio had seen a pattern that told a whole story.
>
> "How did you see that?" I asked, shaking my head. "How'd you find it?"
>
> "Camera is ..." Michio shrugged and pursed his lip to show that he was thinking deeply. "Camera sees only a small piece of what your mind sees." [...].
>
> "If you look into the camera, your mind fools what you see. Maybe ... look at what camera really sees".
>
> "But you've made something from nothing here".
>
> "No, no. This is ..." He paused to get the words right, then carefully pronounced every syllable: "A picture should make you think about a story". (Schooler, 2002, pp. 22–27)

Commentary

What the protagonist of the novel describes is a concrete fact, i.e., observing a photo picture. This experience somehow "captures" his soul. Some of the elements of nature which he knows well from a scientific point of view, seen/grasped by the eye of the artist/photographer in a particular mutual relationship and spatial arrangement, plunge deeply into his internal world, mysteriously sparking off his imagination: something of what he sees through the viewfinder of his camera, because of its aesthetic qualities of balance and dynamism, takes the shape of a dream within him. In this way, something important about his mental life becomes visible and knowable. What is, initially, only a vague feeling of awe and surprise, through the upward movement of the eyes, from the inside of the frame to the outside, becomes the "dream" of a mother holding her child into her arms. In this moment, on the basis of a particular aesthetic sensibility, a congruence is created between the external world of nature, as perceived by the eye of the artist/photographer, and the self-expression of the protagonist of the novel.

Reverie

Mrs F was intent on observing her baby, born premature and weighing a little more than a kilogram. He was lying in his incubator, all covered with wires; his mouth was twisted because of the tube of the respirator, and was immobilised by soft cushions on each side of his head. Suddenly, she said to the nurse next to her that Luca, her baby, was really "a little rascal". Two days earlier, the baby, maybe inadvertently, had removed his respirator with his tiny hand. The nurse was quite struck by the mother's remark, and she wondered how she could call him "a little rascal". She thought that the baby looked not very viable and quite suffering, not yet "a real baby" in many ways. The following week, the same nurse met the mother in front of the incubator of the "little rascal"; meanwhile, he had been detached from the respirator, and was able to move freely. She immediately noticed that the baby, unlike the previous time, was particularly restless, moving quickly and jerkily, "moving all over the place". At the same time, she also noticed that he was able to grasp his mother's finger as soon as it was offered to him, and that he did it with so much strength that his tiny hand became white for the effort. In doing so, however, he became quite calm. The nurse pointed this out to the mother, who smiled with great joy. Unfortunately, this enchanted moment was soon interrupted by the baby sneezing twice. The mother quickly withdrew her hand from the incubator and decided to close its portholes for fear that her baby might feel cold. At this point, the baby started moving agitatedly once again, but he kept his tiny hand, which had grasped his mother's finger outstretched towards the side of the incubator where his mother stood. A few moments later she opened the two portholes once again, and the baby immediately stuck his hand out of the opening. The mother noticed this, smiled, and as she offered her finger for him to grasp, she said to the nurse: "Do you see that he is a little rascal?" The baby held on to his mother's finger and finally began to look at her.

Commentary

Just as in the previous situation the eye of the artist/photographer, supported by his particular aesthetic sensibility, was able to compose a picture of the natural landscape of Alaska in the form of a "story", here, the eyes of a mother, thanks to her maternal capacity for reverie, are able to grasp a particular psychic quality in her prematurely born baby, which is invisible to us. The photographic frame and the mother's image of the baby give shape to something that transcends what the scientific eye of the explorer can see, despite his vast knowledge of petrified forests, and of the nurse, despite her study of the "facts" of medicine; indeed, they establish an intimate and profound link between two people—the photographer and the explorer, the mother and her baby—based on the acknowledgement that what the observer is able to see, in you or for you, somehow belongs to you and allows your Self to find its true expression.

The gathering of the transference

At this point I would like to discuss the first three assessment meetings with Richard (R), a seven-year-old boy, with the purpose of following, step by step, the unfolding of his internal world, his phantasies, his anxieties and defences within the therapeutic relationship. This is a fundamental process of the therapeutic work with children, which Dr Meltzer (1967) called "the gathering of the transference". In this way, you will be able to witness the first transformation of the child's initial symptomatic behaviour into images, feelings, and shared mental contents.

Even after years of work, I am still amazed to see prematurely how, in not so disturbed patients like R, this process gets started in an almost "natural" way. The impression is that of taking part in a very beautiful event, which is the result of the coming together of the incessant need of the child's mind to find transference objects in external reality, and of the beauty of the psychoanalytical method, that offers a sufficiently intimate and safe space within which the child can externalise his internal world, even in its most painful aspects, just as it happens in the relationship between a mother and her baby.

In this context you will see how my "participation" in the analytical experience, on one hand, takes the form of an effort to make R reflect on the emotional significance of certain aspects of his behaviour with his real parents; and on the other, to find, with him and for him, by paying more attention to his communications, both verbal and non-verbal, an imaginative language that can give shape to his infantile emotions in a more personal and unique manner, thus fostering their maturation. What we will observe in these three meetings with a neurotic child might often take years of hard analytic work with more seriously ill patients, and sometimes only in a very limited and partial way. For this reason it is very painful to meet autistic or psychotic children, who are not able to come alive, *vis-à-vis* the emotional experience of the intimacy of an object relationship.

I meet R for the first time towards the end of his second year of primary school, when he is about six and a half years old. He is the only son. His mother works in the field of information technology and his father is a house builder. At birth, his immature respiratory system caused him serious asphyxia, and he was immediately hospitalised in an intensive therapy unit, where he remained for several weeks.

In his early infancy, R had serious difficulties in eating and in his sleep-wake rhythms, which were later overcome, with great effort and patience on everybody's part, when he started going to school. Later, he appeared to be a difficult child in his relationship with the other children, being unable to express positive feelings towards them, whom he approaches with a provocative and annoying attitude.

The parents, desperate, confused, and overwhelmed by his tyrannical behaviour decided to ask for help. R does not tolerate his mother's silence in his presence; he cannot bear her being absorbed in her silent thoughts, especially when the two of them are in the car. He attacks her, urgently demanding her to speak or sing. He grasps her face with his hands, pressing her cheeks to turn her on. "Sing! Sing! Sing!", he screams repeatedly. If she tries to resist he becomes furious, starts crying and screaming, accusing her of being a bad mother, and even slaps and kicks her, if he can. He is exhausting and violent, and there is no way of convincing him of the meaninglessness of his behaviour.

R is tyrannical also with his father, whom he puts to the test asking him for constant "acts of love". In the evening, when it is time to go to bed, he demands his father to fall asleep next to his bed; in the morning, upon awakening, he runs (if he hasn't already done so in the middle of the night) to his parents' bed, steals his mother's place who is forced to go into another room, and when the time comes to wake up, he is the one that wants to turn the alarm clock off and decide his father's schedule, detaining him for a long time on the threshold of the bathroom with a never ending request for kisses ... and if, during the day, the father phones home and he suspects that the phone-call isn't only for him, but also for his mother, he immediately interrupts the conversation and has him call back.

First meeting

He arrives with his mother. He follows her to the steps that lead to the entrance of my office, slightly hidden behind her. He is looking at her and it looks as if he is begging her to not leave him with me. He is a small child, amiable, dressed in a sporty, accurate way. He seems to have just got out of school. His haircut is short.

I say hello to him and he looks into my eyes. He has a curious expression, not distressed, a bit adult-like. I invite him to come into the bright playroom in front of us, lit up by the light of the window that gives on to a small garden, while I ask his mother to wait in the waiting room. I make him understand that his mother is waiting for him in there. He does not seem to give much importance to what I say. He follows me and sits down, in an orderly fashion, on the chair next to the side of the table, on one of the long walls of the room, near the window. I sit in front of him on the other side of the table. He looks at me in silence. In this short silent pause we hear some banging on the floor coming from the apartment upstairs and the rustling of the dry magnolia leaves on the cobbled paving of the courtyard downstairs. R, alarmed, takes note of these noises but does not say anything. He notices a mosquito buzzing around me. He quickly gets up and in a flash captures and kills it. He sits back down on the chair, in a very orderly fashion, and silent as before.

Some more noises are heard from the upstairs apartment and from outside. R, initially alarmed, asks me what they are, and then gets up and looks out of the window to see if there is anyone in the garden. He sits down again. He continues to look into my eyes. He doesn't seem anxious, it actually seems as if he's waiting for me to guide our conversation. At this point I ask him why he came to me. After a brief pause, with my help, he finally tells me that he often argues with his mother, when he is in the car he commands her because her silence irritates him. He hates the fact that she is mute. In addition, he says that he also commands his dad. At night, before going to bed, he wants his father to stay near his bed until he falls asleep and wants him to be there in the morning as well.

While telling me about these things he uses a normal tone of voice, without any trace of anxiety or emotion. It sounds as if he wants to tell me: "That's the way it is, what do you want to do about it, it's not a problem! They're not important things, they're annoying at the most." He does not seem to be able to understand the emotional impact that his behaviour has on his parents. He minimises.

[…]

He looks at the open toy box on the table and all of a sudden he tells me that he has an idea. He wants to do a drawing, a drawing of a spider (Drawing 1). He takes a black marker and a white sheet of paper and starts sketching in one of the corners a spider's web that has in the middle a ball of lines that represent a prey. Then he draws a vertical line, to which he hangs the spider. He's precise and meticulous in tracing the body and the head of the animal, but then, as he draws the first two legs, he does on, which is not in proportion to the other one. He tells me that he has made a mistake. He seems disappointed and worried. He would like to immediately correct the wrong leg, eliminate it with some correcting fluid, but he is scared that he might make an even worse mess. He is very tense, as if he were in front of a real drama. He seems not to know what to do. I invite him to start his drawing over on another piece of paper (Drawing 2). He accepts my suggestion. He starts a new drawing in which he traces a kind of confused web in the top left corner of the paper and does a nice black spider, with eight legs, a red head with four eyes and two stings with a red tip, completely hanging in the air, without a thread tying him to his web. In the meantime he talks to me about his passion for spiders, even the poisonous ones. At a certain point he notices that while making the spider's web he drew out of the sheet of paper and soiled the table with some black colour. He immediately gets agitated when he sees the dirty table, he looks at me a few times, he does not know what to do, would like to clean everything at once. It is time to say goodbye, and I tell him. Without having to ask him, R puts back his things in the box. While he is leaving the room, he tells me that the next time he will come accompanied by his father.

Commentary

In this first meeting I am impressed by the indifference that the child shows towards me at the beginning, and that he also shows towards the pain that his tyrannical behaviour generates in his parents, and by the intense, insistent anxiety that he feels when he is struck by the noises that violently interrupt his silence in the room, *and when he notices he drew one of the spider's legs wrongly and then to have soiled the table.*

Second meeting

He arrives accompanied by his father. With him he has a bag of crunchy potato chips already open. He quickly goes into the playroom, while his father sits in the waiting room. I join him and I find him sitting in the same chair that he was on the last time he came. He looks into my eyes as if to say hello or have me greet him. He is very hungry and eats the potato chips with pleasure and voracity.

[…]

I decide to talk to him right away about an idea that came to mind while pondering on the conversations we had in our last meeting about the spider. I tell him that I am surprised and a little puzzled that I found out that while he makes everyone believe, especially his mother and his father, that he is a very fragile and distressed child, he has told me that he has no fear of spiders or of the dark; in fact, he has repeatedly told me that spiders are his favourite animals, even the dangerous and poisonous ones. "So—I add with a playful tone of voice—your being the 'commander' with mum and dad maybe has not got anything to do with the fact that you are a scared child, but rather with the fact that you want to control your mother and your father, keep them separate and always busy with you … who knows, maybe they have in mind to give you a little brother?"

R answers me with ease, as if he were talking of something obvious, that he does not want brothers, that it is true that he commands and controls his parents to prevent them from having another child. I notice that while he is telling me these things he does not let any potato chip get caught in his throat. So I ask him if he knows how babies are born. With the look of one that does not want to think about it, he answers me that we know that, "It's God who wants them". With some effort he adds that maybe "Also some cuddling is involved". In the meantime he has finished the chips. He gets up to throw away the coloured plastic paper in the basket and puts on the table the surprise that he has found in the bag of potato chips. Then he sits down once again.

After a short pause, still staring at my face, he says that he has thought of a drawing. He gets everything he needs to write, paper, a pencil, pastel colours, and adhesive tape. He divides the sheet of paper in two parts with a line; above it, he draws and colours a fish with a red tail, covered with scales, and below it, a parrot with a light blue body, closed inside a frame (Drawing 3). Then he hides the drawing of the two animals under a strip of adhesive tape and he explains: "In this way the colour does not get ruined." I think that maybe the fish and the bird represent in his mind the father and mother we are talking about, they are two images of mom and dad, that he wants to protect, but that he keeps apart, as the line traced in the middle of the sheet of paper shows. R pretends not to listen. All of a sudden he puts his drawing away, saying that it is "dirty". I carefully look at the drawing and all I can see are some pencil smudges that do not spoil it at all. Instead I think that his anxiety about the dirt has to do with his infantile sadistic anal phantasies towards his parents.

While I am thinking about this, R takes another sheet of paper (Drawing 4) and, hiding behind the box, he quickly draws another picture, with two paintings on the left; the first one on top, represents a fishing trophy, while the one at the bottom a hunting trophy: the same mother-fish as before, pierced by a harpoon, and the father-bird with a hole caused by a bullet. I see the drawing only when it is finished. It is actually R that shows it to me with a look of understanding. During this time we keep talking about how babies are born. "We left off at the cuddles", I remind him. While drawing, R tells me with a slight "know-it-all" attitude that he knows everything about the fish and the birds, he was taught by a fisherman and a hunter, who were his friends. He tells me, for example, that he knows how to perfectly distinguish if a fish is male or female, from its colour. His lesson on sea breams, soles, basses, and on their sexual differences, does not seem very illuminating. I interrupt him, saying that he, too, seems now closer to believing that besides God and cuddles, also sex and genitals are involved in the making of a baby.

He needs to poo. He runs to the bathroom from which he returns after a while, after having done everything by himself. Sitting on the chair he starts asking me if I am a psychologist, if other children come to me as well. Mainly, he insists on knowing if this is my home, and if the analytic couch is the bed where I sleep in after he has gone, with whom I sleep, who is the doctor that he met in the office for a brief moment the last time he came. I tell him that he would like to know many things about me, everything about the fish and the birds or how he would like to know everything that is in his mother's head when she is quiet.

I explain to him that I am only going to answer some of his questions. I am going to answer him in a way that I know is not going to interfere with our job. I do not tell him anything about the other children. I specify that the house in which I live in is in another area of the city and that the doctor is my wife. I add that I was impressed with the quickness with which he imagined that the playroom becomes the room where we grownups sleep at night.

The hour is finished. I remind him that we still have another meeting on the same day at the same hour, like today. R does not stand up and not seem to be in a rush to leave. Before leaving, though, he does something else: he takes the surprise gift he found in the bag of potato chips, a "gooey character", and he sticks it to the wall of the room.

Commentary

R starts letting himself get involved in the exploration of the infantile transference primarily towards his original objects, his parents, and partially towards the therapeutic situation. The child turns out to be interested in certain subjects and his mind works in an associative way. It is clear that the observations I make on his behaviour, on the details of his drawings, on his relationship with dirt, are heavily influenced by the Kleinian theories of early object relations and of primitive anxiety situations. While I carry out this exploratory routine job, I am aware of the existence of a big communication problem with the child, which would require something more inspired, particularly in the use of language and images.

Third meeting

Today R arrives with his mother fifteen minutes early, so he takes a seat in the waiting room where I go to get him at his hour. Once we are in the room he immediately sits in his chair and remains in silence for a few minutes keeping his eyes on me. When I ask him if he is thinking of something, he answers that he is not thinking of anything. So I suggest we look at his drawings together. I take them out of the folder one by one in chronological order, I look at them carefully, and I repeat to him what I had already told him in the last session, talking about his need to control mum and dad since he does not want any little siblings to be born. He listens to me very carefully but does not seem to want to resume thinking about these topics. He keeps silent for a few minutes, and then with a start he tells me that he has thought of another picture, but I must not see.

He builds a barrier with the toy box and some toys, behind which he hides to escape from my sight. Then he gets the drawing material ready.

I am surprised when R starts pulling out from underneath his sweater with slow, cautious movements, a big black compressed-air toy gun. He places it on the sheet of paper without making any noise and starts outlining it. Pleased with the result, he does the same thing on another sheet of paper. Now and then he takes his eyes off the table, he stops to raise the walls of his hiding place with some toys. He looks at me with an "insolent" look that makes me smile. Maybe this makes him understand that I can actually see everything through the transparent box. So he grabs the gun, and holding it firmly with both hands he points it at me so I can see it well. I am stunned by the size of the weapon in comparison to his small child hands. He tells me that the gun is a present from his mother, a prize for the good report card he received at the end of the school year. I suggest that maybe he came armed to this session since he is not convinced that this place is really quite safe.

While I'm talking with the child I think of a hunter in the middle of the jungle that, after having shot his prey, for a few minutes, in the surreal silence that follows the pistol shot, lives with fear that the animal is just wounded and could jump on him at any time. I immediately associate this image with the anxiety that Richard feels about his silent mother.

R makes me notice that the pistol magazine is empty because he left the plastic bullets at home. He then starts loading the pistol. He first inserts the pencil in the gun barrel. He tries to shoot but he fails. The pencil is too heavy. Then with scissors he starts making smaller and lighter bullets. He cuts the pointy end of the crayons. He breaks the pencil into several parts as well and takes the lead out. He then attempts some other ballistic strategies with new bullets. He shoots several times in my direction but towards the more distant corner of my chair, where the rubbish bin is, then, pleased with the results, he gradually starts aiming at me. I make him notice this and suggest that maybe he is aiming at me because he does not trust his doctor, either. Almost to reassure or to calm me he clarifies that it is a toy gun, not a real one like dad's, which he uses to protect himself when he goes to work!

He needs to poo. He runs to the bathroom and like the previous sessions he does everything by himself. When he comes back he asks whose was the female voice he heard coming from the room near the bathroom, inside which he had peeked at the end of our second meeting. I answer him saying that it is the voice of a doctor that works with me in the office. He immediately asks me if the bed that is in the room is where the doctor and I sleep in at night. He concentrates on making new bullets.

While cutting the tip of the brown crayon he notices that there is some dirt left on one of the scissor blades. He examines it carefully. Then he comes close to me and shows it to me saying that it looks like the profile of three people, of a mother, and a father with a child. It looks like a sculpture, thin as a drawing or as a comic strip. Then he grabs the piece of paper with the first drawing of the gun, he makes it into a ball and starts throwing it towards the rubbish bin, trying to get it into the basket. He makes three or four throws and then stops because he notices that the other drawing of the gun and the table are smudged with the coloured pastel dust and the black pencil lead. Worried, he looks at the mess that he has made, but he does not do anything either to save his drawing or to tidy up or clean the table.

He proceeds to shoot other bullets in the air towards the rubbish bin, more and more excited; finally, he puts a bullet in his mouth, waiting for my comment or rebuke. He sucks it with greed, pretending to like the piece of coloured crayon. I remain silent. R keeps sucking, until he spits it out disgusted, but to his great disappointment he does not manage this easily, because the bullet remains stuck to his lips. Once he has managed to clean his mouth, not without difficulties, he continues shooting at the rubbish bin from his chair with his gun. After every shot he stands up to retrieve the bullet, which he puts back into the gun barrel for the next shot and goes back to his initial position. I observe in silence what he does. At a certain point he stops to ask me what the two parallel lines which run down the two sides of the gun and reach the tip are. I explain to him that they are the marks that help you aim well.

After a while he stops shooting and comes near me, putting the gun into my hands and asking me to shoot. I refuse. R insists in his request. I realise that he is playing a joke on me. I keep refusing to shoot. At a certain point R gives up and shows me that the trigger is blocked because there is a safety lock. I look at the gun and I check that it is actually blocked. I am very impressed by his interest in the safety lock of the gun and I think that he is looking for a paternal function that can make his relationships safer and more protected.

Moving closer to him, I tell him that I have noticed that he really likes to be a strong and powerful hunter, but maybe in certain moments there is another that feels scared like a little bird or a little fish, looking for protection. It is the end of the hour. At my signal that we have to say goodbye, R reacts with a shudder, as if he had been shot. Out of the room he asks his mom if he can bring me a fish, which he caught. The mother looks at me, confused, as if to ask, "Should I?", and she tells me that R is particularly fond of fishing. I tell the child that there is no need for him to bring his fish to me; next time, instead, we will try to understand the meaning of his request.

Commentary

At the end of the third meeting there is a change in the way the child is present in my imagination. Like the mother of the premature baby, or like the Japanese photographer, I find him inside me through an image, that of the hunter in the jungle, which has the quality of a dream thought. Some present iconographic aspects can be easily referred to my direct observations of the child, but overall they are composed in such a way as to narrate a story, or even better, many stories, depending on the meaning that we want to attribute to them.

I immediately realise that the image is full of elements and important links (as we saw before in the case of the image of the "little rascal" and of the photograph) which allow me to reflect on the patient's infantile transference in a more realistic way, less explicative, and to place his tyrannical behaviour toward his mother's silence in a narrative, non-causal dimension. There is a very interesting spatial element, the "being inside the jungle", that represents the inside of the mother's body, and in a broader sense, life in general: an extreme place, where the child is powerful and terrorised at the same time, both hunter and potential victim. Not a place for pleasant meetings, without tension. It can be thought as the world in which he has been projected at birth, as his experience in the incubator in the intensive therapy unit.

The silence of the jungle, like the silence of the mother, becomes the signal that somewhere, invisible potential enemies are hidden, whose presence can be revealed only by the rustling of the grass or the plunk of a branch that breaks (I think of R's anxiety for the rustling of the leaves coming from my garden and the thuds on the floor from upstairs). For the child there is something unsaid or inexpressible, secretly dangerous, which lives in the mind of adults.

With some help from this image, I feel I can talk to the child not only of his identity as a strong and powerful hunter, but also of his hunter's fears, and above all, of his anxiety of being the victim of an evil hunter or fisherman. It is not easy to talk to him about how much he is distressed, while he is pacing around the therapy room armed, even if I am led in this direction by the theme of "the gun's safe", but this is made possible by the integration of these two polarities of his experience of identity in my story, where the hunter that kills his prey immediately fears its revenge; the hunter that feels strong and powerful with his gun is the same person that does not know what is hidden behind the silence following the shot.

Sleep without dreams

Alongside the clinical situations that I have just described, in which the careful and detailed observation of the child's behaviour and play activity leads to the understanding of its significance and emotional value, there are others in which the therapist experiments a total (or almost total) inability to identify himself with his patients. This happens in psychotherapeutic and psychoanalytic work with children and young adolescents suffering from a generalised developmental disorder, during which the therapist has to deal with primitive, dramatic countertransference experiences, characterised by a sudden alteration of his attention and consensual capacity, which make him "plunged" into a dreamless sleep, and by the difficulty of having "dream thoughts" about the events that are maturing within the analytic relationship. In the therapist and his patients there is a total inability to get access to shared meanings, and for long periods of time they all live in their own solipsism.

I would now like to discuss the notes concerning a therapy session with Alessio (Al), a sixteen-year-old boy suffering from Asperger's Syndrome, in his tenth year of therapy. It is interesting material since the patient, *urged by the imminent end of his treatment, in a few months' time,* seems to be in the process of discovering that there is a "soul" in things, and he seems to be wondering about important issues, such as life before birth and the pain of separation. Apparently, his arguments seem pertinent; however, one can notice that he is unable to organise the notions available to him so as to allow emotions to be expressed: he produces beliefs, built on a causal chain of events, and pseudo-scientific theories, like the transmigration of the soul, whose aim is to keep emotions at a distance, rather than express them, to which it is difficult to latch on, if not in a didactic, conclusive manner. He tries to get an idea about sadness by drawing tears on his face; or he tries to decide who of us is bigger, who must command and have more authority, on the basis of our respective heights.

Al arrives alone, with the lift. His hands are quite busy, as usual, with the ice cream, the tissue to wipe his lips with, and his sweater. He is nervous. He gets a bit angry with the lift door, which does not close automatically, and then he comes in the therapy room and sits down. Immediately, without looking at me, he says to me: "I would like to tell you …" He is angry because he does not remember, despite his efforts, the place where his soul was before 1988, the year of his birth.

He repeats several times, in a confused way, that it would have been better if he had been an Australopithecus for two years, and then become a "*Homo sapiens*" when he was born. Today, he would like to know from me (he wants to have a "precise answer") where his soul was before 1988; he wants to know the exact place. He would like to have a time machine. He imagines he can build one (he tells me that nothing is impossible, as long as one has all the "materials" available …).

I talk to him about the world of the mind, about the things that belong to the world of the imagination and of those that belong to reality. Then he turns to GOD, looking outside the window, as if the soul might be somewhere in the sky/heaven, only God knows where. Then, after listening to my words (I try to make him think that we are not immortal, that we are born only the moment when our parents begin to want a baby and then, with their intercourse, their idea is made flesh), he defines his own theory, saying that he once was inside the primitive, hairy body of an "Australopithecus" (a bit worried, he tells me that the primitive man threw stones at the evil animals, chasing them away; he did not want them near him—he seems to be talking about his infantile part, jealous and frightened of the other children). Then he melted the body of the primitive man in brine, and his white soul (like a ghost, let's hope mummy did not see it, otherwise she might be scared) entered into his mother's body and was embodied in the child she carried inside her. Then "I was born, I sucked her milk …". He is convinced that if we do not remember the place where we were before being born it is because we were blind. I try to make him understand that his exact theory about his origins is also the fruit of his imagination, of his mind. He also tells me that when he was born they gave him the first name Al "because, before that, only his surname was known". He looks outside the window, because he has seen a flash (there is a thunderstorm outside).

[….]

Towards the end of the session I make him notice how he has changed in the past few weeks, his interests have become more profound, and we both feel that the time available to us is really very little. I talk to him about the sad shadow I see in his eyes towards the end of our sessions. He bides his time playing "strike", trying to throw a rubber ball into a basket.

As he leaves the room, he compares his height to mine, saying that he is almost as tall as me, even if that is not true. He insists on wanting to be right, as if to reverse a painful situation, a deep feeling of inferiority and inadequacy. He goes to the bathroom. I look inside and I see that he is washing his face, dabbing his eyes (with a wet paper tissue). He dries his face, and then he wets his eyes again (tears, makeup?). To interrupt his rituals I raise the tone of my voice a bit. He moves near me and with a challenging—but tender—expression, he asks me if I am reprimanding him. I tell him that I do not want him to get lost in his rituals, since our time is precious. Immediately after that, as if to placate me, he comes nearer to me, once again compares our heights and calmly acknowledges that I am taller than him.

Commentary

Al thinks and deals with his worries as he does with the idea of a time machine that he is convinced he can build it. "It is just a matter of 'materials'", he says. He believes that a solution to them is easily accessible. There is no need of "imagination". He shows me that he still does not have an internal function able to assemble/construct the elements that are available to him—his observations on reality—in a symbol, in a dream thought, in a scientific hypothesis. Moreover, these notes do not show the natural enfolding, in the analytic relationship, of an internal world full of transference meanings, as we saw in the case of Riccardo. There is something that is still "missing" in Al's internal landscape: infantile emotional life.

The language of poetry

The session with Al clearly shows the difficulties we might encounter with seriously ill patients when we try to describe what happens within the analytic relationship in order to spark off their imagination. On one side there is my patient, who wants to have "precise" answers about "ineffable topics": he wants to know exactly where he was before he was born, exactly how many centimetres are needed to be considered a "grownup", what is the exact trick to be able to show your sadness to the others; while I am on the other side, trying to survive his siege, to avoid his quizzing questions by providing him with informative answers, still unable to organise my observations—internal and external—in a transcription, a notation, a pattern, a dream thought that might support/promote the symbolic transformation of his concrete reasoning.

You might well ask, then, what can come to the therapist's aid, at that point. I think that, in such moments, only poetry and art in general can help a therapist understand what it is that prevents the interests of his patient from becoming "experience". For this reason, I would like to invite you to read two poems by Rabindranath Tagore (1903, 1916), which deal with the same themes present in the session I have just reported, with the eyes and the language of a poet.

The beginning (1916)

> "Where have I come from, where did you pick me up?" the baby asked its mother.
>
> She answered half crying, half laughing, and clasping the baby to her breast,—"You were hidden in my heart as its desire, my darling.
>
> You were in the dolls of my childhood's games; and when with clay I made the image of my god every morning, I made and unmade you then.
>
> You were enshrined with our household deity, in his worship I worshipped you.
>
> In all my hopes and my loves, in my life, in the life of my mother you have lived.
>
> In the lap of the deathless Spirit who rules our home you have been nursed for ages.
>
> When in girlhood my heart was opening its petals, you hovered as a fragrance about it.
>
> Your tender softness bloomed in my youthful limbs, like a glow in the sky before the sunrise.
>
> Heaven's first darling, twin-born with the morning light, you have floated down the stream of the world's life, and at last you have stranded on my heart.
>
> As I gaze on your face, mystery overwhelms me; you who belong to all have become mine.
>
> For fear of losing you I hold you tight to my breast. What magic has snared the world's treasure in these slender arms of mine?"
>
> (Tagore, 1913)

Death of the child (1903)

It was alive, it laughed,
it walked and played.
Nature, what did you get when you took it?
You have millions of coloured birds,
Forests, stars, oceans,
The infinite sky.
Why did you tear it away from its mother's breast,
Hid it in the earth's womb
And covered it with flowers?
O mighty Nature,
Of thousands of stars and flowers,
You have stolen a child!
Has your infinite treasure
Been enriched by this, perhaps?
Has your happiness increased
By a tiny speck?
And yet, a mother's heart,
As boundless as yours,
With the loss of her child
Has lost everything!
(Tagore, *Morte del bambino*, 1903 [1979])

Commentary

What strikes me in these two poems is mainly the poet's ability to identify himself with a mother's joy or sorrow. Tagore seems to "know" the intensity of the feelings that make a child appear so "precious" to its mother's eyes. He speaks about the birth of a baby as a gift of life, and of its death as an unjust and incomprehensible misappropriation brought about by some greedy force of nature He seems to be saying that the child is "precious" because it belongs to something that transcends maternal feelings; it has a "divine" origin in the eternity of time, and once it has been born—even in its death—it belongs to the wonders of nature. Therefore, it is precious because it is part of the "mystery" of life, to which a mother—by means of her child—seems to have access more than any other being. The feelings of joy and sorrow, the love, as well as the hate of life, which takes the child away with death, are put at the service of the wish for knowledge and are removed from the dangers of romantic agony and cynicism. In these poems, the birth and death of a child become the opportunity to reconsider the feeling of "awe/wonder" which our soul experiences every time it is exposed to the mystery of life and death, or rather, to the mystery of the beauty of life and its fragility. And among the beautiful, mysterious and fascinating things in life there are also the processes that characterise the birth and the development of a child's mind.

In the light of all this, we might ask ourselves what Al is trying to communicate to us with his pseudo-scientific accounts of his origins, of his life before birth, or with his "game" in front of the bathroom mirror, when he seemed to rehearse his crying and make himself up like a sad clown before appearing on a stage. Maybe he started to feel that our link has become precious—because of some mysterious "alchemy"—and that this makes our separation/parting complicated and possibly painful?

Final remarks

Before concluding, I would like to understand if the examples of interaction between the eyes and the mind, which I have just presented to you, might also offer further opportunities to clarify and develop some of the considerations that I mentioned in my introduction, where I pointed out the need for the analyst to deeply modify his observational stance, because of the severity of the psychopathological situations he has to deal with. A general remark I made was that the observation of the child should be informed by a less tense and more extended attention, and accompanied by a different sort of receptivity, free from theories and explanatory statements.

Reading the two pages from Lynn Schooler's book *The Blue Bear* was of great interest to me; in fact, apart from reminding us how important art can be in favouring the contact with our emotions and their expression—the interest we have in our emotional experiences and their meaning is not a natural thing for our mental apparatus, which is more predisposed to action rather than self-consciousness—it shows us how the eyes of the artist/photographer, guided by a great love for nature and by a particular aesthetic sensibility, can notice some connections between the physical elements in nature, some movements that, as a whole, make up an object (the photograph), the beauty of which captures the attention of those who observe it, bringing forth feelings and thoughts that have to do with the knowledge we have of ourselves and of the world, with the revelation of ourselves and the world.

For the child, also the mother is an object of great aesthetic attraction, and *vice versa,* and doubtlessly this mutual attraction is fundamental for the development of a good mother-child relationship. The material from my second example has always fascinated me also for another reason linked to the theme of the receptivity of the analyst's mind and of the value of his observations in support of his interpretations. How is it that the eyes of a mother can see in her child something that we either cannot see at all, or can only see belatedly? What guarantees do we have that what a mother sees in her child is true? In order to understand this situation it would be appropriate to think, as Bion (1962) suggested, that the mother has a particular skill in getting in touch with the psychic qualities of her child: the maternal capacity for reverie. Hence, we must be aware of the importance of increasing—through our observational studies—our capacity for reverie and for the acknowledgement of the psychic qualities of a child's experience.

The third example, linked to the clinical case of Richard, helps us discover two important dimensions of the therapist's observational function. The first is similar to the flight of migratory birds: it is a careful, accurate, watchful, selective in terms of the details of the child's behaviour and the contents of its play activity and communications; it is guided by the therapist's particular sensibility towards the psychic qualities of the child's experiences (a sort of maternal reverie, or internal radar) and by his own theoretical knowledge, and it aims at favouring the gathering and evolution of the infantile transference within the analytic situation (Meltzer, 1967) (the flight destination) as well as its acknowledgement.

The second is an observation which tries to grasp the qualitative aspects of the verbal and non-verbal inter subjective communications between the child and the analyst; it is supported by the therapist's particular sensibility towards the compositional aspects of intersubjective communication (which is equivalent to the aesthetic sensibility of the eye of the artist/photographer towards the natural landscape). In the fourth and fifth example we are faced with two very different personalities: a young adolescent suffering from Asperger's syndrome and a poet, Tagore; both of them are struggling with an important question, the same question that the baby asks its mother in Tagore's first poem: "Where have I come from?" In the first case, the answer found by the patient confirms the tragic blindness of his eyes; whereas the answer found by the poet reveals an act of seeing which is supported by his passion for life, going deep down in the world of emotions, and then bringing to the surface—and making them visible also to those who did not know they possessed them—"those secrets that remain indecipherable to us" (Ungaretti, 1916).

Drawings

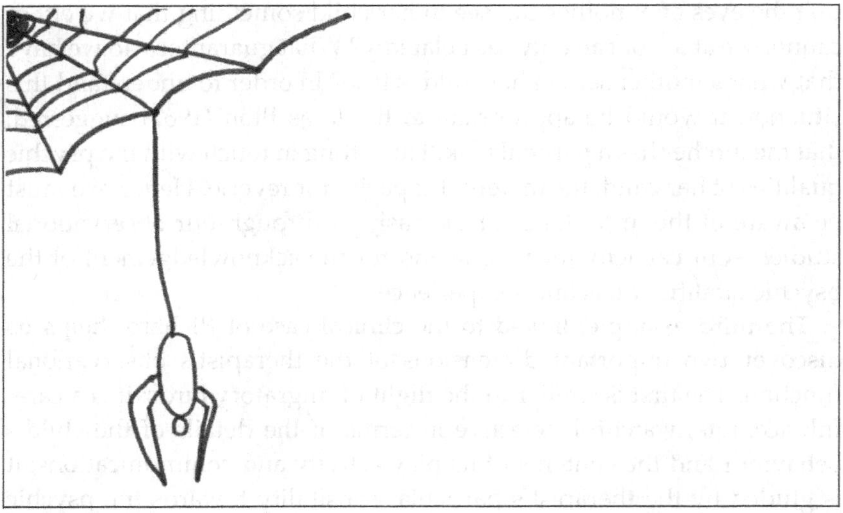

Drawing 1. Spider and web.

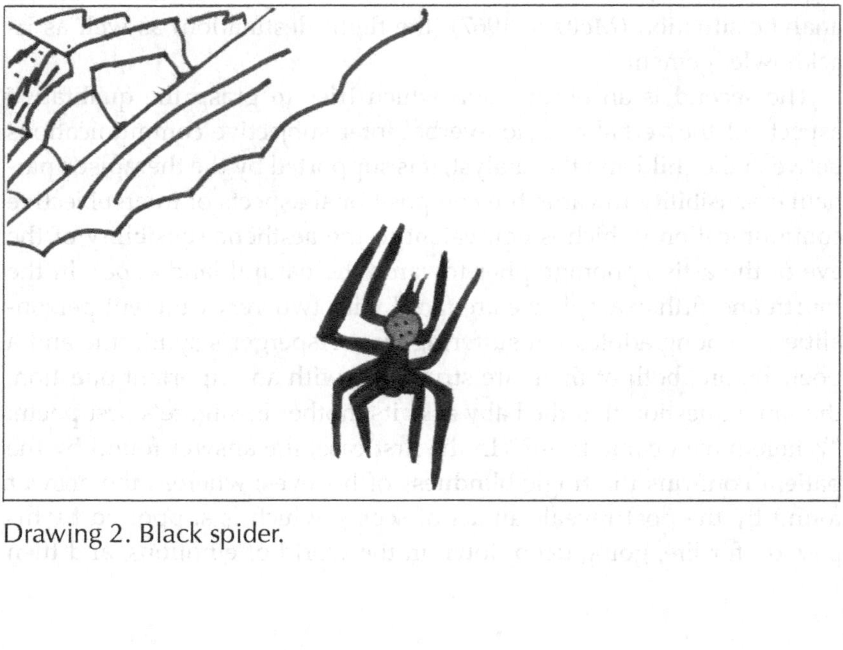

Drawing 2. Black spider.

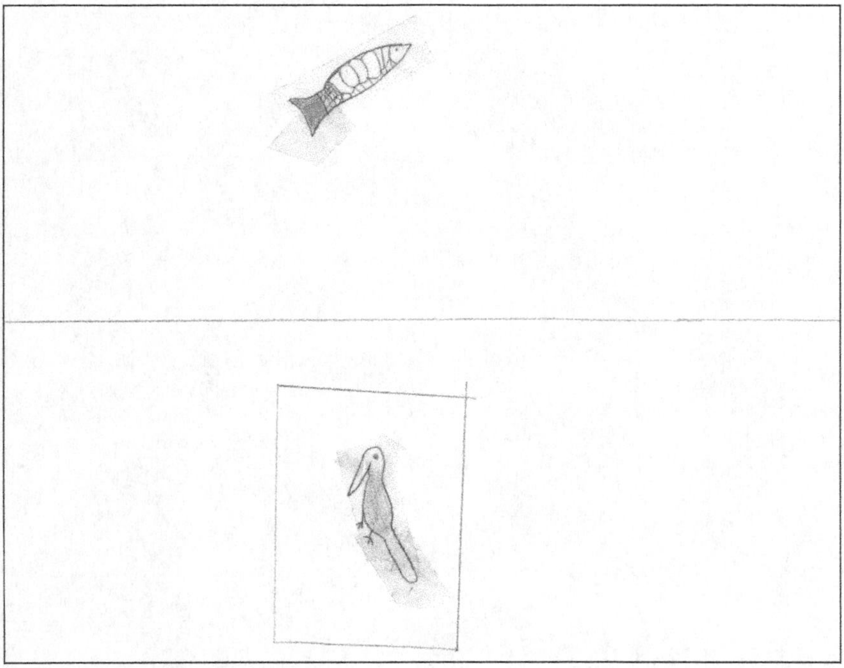

Drawing 3. Fish and parrot.

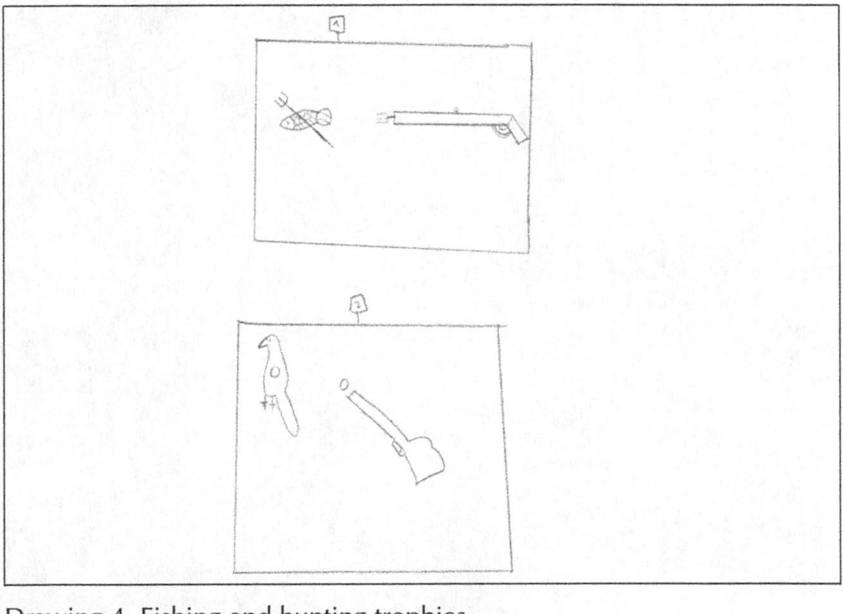

Drawing 4. Fishing and hunting trophies.

PART II

CLINICAL FINDINGS

CHAPTER FOUR

What can be done if the mind does not develop? Encountering bi-dimensionality and absence of meaning while working with child and adolescent psychotics*

Introduction

In the course of our work as psychoanalysts of children and adolescents, we have found that in recent years there has been a steady increase in the number of psychotic patients suffering from serious delay in the structuring of their personality, with peculiar character traits and social and intellectual limitations mainly due to a failure to enter a three-dimensional world in their mental life rather than with a state of confusion in their sense of identity. Their internal world was flat, populated with few fragmented and degraded objects with no emotional light. Their relationship with others and with the emotions they give rise to was based mainly on automatic mechanisms of consent or dissent, or on mechanisms of avoidance and closure of an autistic type.

---

*This chapter is a modified version of a text that was read for at the First Conference of the Italian Section of the EFPP (Rome, 27th–29th January 1995), and then published by Bertolini, R. & Caccia, O. in *Richard & Piggle, 2/96*, pp. 164–182, Il *Pensiero Scientifico Editore*. The co-author, Mrs Ornella Caccia is a psychoanalytic psychotherapist for children, adolescents, and parents, and teaches in the observational and clinical courses of the AIPPI in Rome and of the CSMH of Florence.

By automatic consent we mean all adhesive ways of relating to others (adhesive identification, adhesive behaviour, adhesive learning); by automatic dissent we mean all negativistic ways of relating to others (negative identification, behaving in the opposite way to that expected such as by laughing when crying or being frightened is expected, or spitting out when drinking is in order, or by saying words with their syllables reversed).

However this study has been stimulated above all, by the discovery that the deep significance of the therapeutic process, as it has developed through constant contact with these patients, could no longer be represented by the literary metaphor of Dante's journey. The analytic relationship with these patients tended to take on rather the meaning of animation or re-animation than the resolution of confusional states or persecutory anxiety, and thus became similar to a dreaming process which aimed at coagulating, protecting, and giving form to primary emotional tensions (proto-emotions) which in their personality had no way of developing into so-called real emotions because they were suffocated at the outset by negativistic behaviour, or avoided through autistic closure, or magically bypassed by an adhesive answer. This took place so quickly to appear like an automatic reaction, and in all three circumstances the patients' attention was removed from the moment of experience and concentrated elsewhere or switched off. Our aim in this study therefore, has been to further explore the concept of bi-dimensionality, which we consider equivalent to the absence of mental life i.e., the alpha-function cannot be set in motion so that symbolic chains cannot be developed, or they are destroyed soon after birth. We have tried to present some considerations on the therapeutic quality required in order to have an effect on this particular type of pathology. The clinical material on which we have based our study has been drawn from the psychotherapy of a boy, Antonio (A), who is now twenty-two years old and who received treatment during adolescence (from fourteen years on) from Dr Bertolini, and from the psychotherapy of a child Vincenzo (V) seen by Mrs Caccia since the age of three to date. He is now nine years old. We would like to add that the observations regarding these two patients have been made possible also by the experience we have gained through our analytical work with numerous similar cases, which have been treated or supervised by us. Naturally this work is based on phenomena connected with the development of the transference, which only the analytical method gives access to. Above all we have referred to what was going on inside the analytic encounter paying attention to those moments which are usually most profound and significant within this relationship, such as entering and leaving the room, the last session before going on holiday, or the first session on return.

Before proceeding with our clinical material we would like to outline some background details of the two patients. We will try to be brief and to highlight those aspects of infancy, which were, in our opinion, most significant.

Some background data on A (Dr B)

A began working with me just after his fourteenth birthday, he was repeating the final year of Middle School for the second time. Before he was five he had already received a diagnosis of "infantile autism with dissociative notes" and had undergone psychoanalytical treatment. This therapeutic experience enabled him to break out of actual autism and allowed him to be accepted into the normal education system for young children, where he was constantly assisted by a Special Needs Teacher. In school he was able to learn the basic skills of reading and writing without however developing any particular interest in any subject and above all, without being able to form any relationship with his class mates. He spent much of his time wandering around corridors or chatting with the caretakers or with occasional visitors.

Before taking up therapy again with me A had suspended all forms of treatment over the last two years. As adolescence approached he had begun to manifest serious behavioural difficulties, his tendency to isolate himself had become more accentuated and he had become intensely sexually excitable which led him to masturbate himself in a compulsive and exhibitionistic way. For these reasons and in agreement with the former therapist, he started up therapy again.

Before beginning treatment I had several meetings with A's parents who seemed to be very alarmed by his sexual behaviour and very worried about the exasperating control he seemed to exercise over his sister, two years and eight months younger than him. He tormented her in a thousand ways, touched her genitals and her breasts, and stole her underwear, which he later secretly put on. They told me that he had attacked her by gripping her around the neck from behind.

Talking about A's infancy, his parents told me how good he had been at drawing, and how much pleasure he seemed to get out of it; they underlined however, that he used to be interested only in certain idiosyncratic subjects which for a period dominated all his work in a repetitive and obsessive manner, only to disappear and be replaced by others. There was the period of rivers and fresh water, of roundabouts and of the flight of planes. His parents told me that his drawings were full of "*special perspectives*" (i.e., strange ways of illustrating and describing reality) and that they were very rich in detail. In the same way A was particularly devoted to fairies, and then to princesses, then to ballerinas with tutus which he loved going to see at the theatre, and finally to Barbie dolls. From their accounts a very important aspect of A's character emerges, that of not being able to accept situations, which were different from those he expected or hoped for, whether they represented aspects of daily life, or the interests described above. For example he could not accept his mother cooking without wearing an apron, neither would he tolerate the ballerina wearing a dress that was different from the one he had imagined.

His mother spoke of her experience with A when he was very small. She said that for the first three months A had not given any sign of having difficulty either sleeping or feeding. The first difficulties appeared towards the second half of the first year of his life when she returned to work. The child began to show a progressive and gradual withdrawal from human interaction and his sleeping-waking rhythm was severely disturbed. From vague memories of the first three months of his life the mother gave me a very peculiar description of the child: she told me that A was always trying to follow her everywhere with his eyes, then he would stare at her and move his mouth in her direction as if he wanted to say something to her. She said however, that she was never able to understand what those eyes staring at her meant: there was something odd about it. She concluded that A had always seemed like a Martian to her, meaning that he seemed dangerously foreign.

The father, at those first meetings, told me that when the child was small it was typical of him to oppose any attempt at teaching him anything, such as walking, riding a bike, dressing himself, lacing up his shoes etc. He said that there was always something odd in his attitude towards learning something new, which did not seem connected with fear, at least not apparently. He told me for example, that his first attempts at putting the child on his bike and showing him how to make the correct movements in order to ride without falling off, had met with a strange form of opposition, shown by a passive refusal to carry out the task. The child seemed so inadequate at that point, he decided to stop the lessons for a while. One day, after further vain attempts at teaching his son who let himself passively be pushed around as if he were a rag doll, the father saw him get on the bike and ride round with great skill. When A was older he behaved in the same way when memorising the days of the week and the months of the year. By saying this, the father seemed to confirm the feeling of foreignness and inaccessibility of this son. Furthermore the parents referred to an absolute feeling of exhaustion, which sometimes made them become violent or expulsive. This feeling was related to the fact that A spent long periods worrying them for constant explanations about aspects of daily life that are generally considered as being very marginal, whereas to him these subjects became vitally important and an obsessive preoccupation. He would ask for example, if women could do the same jobs as men, whether old men could marry young women, if he could have a girlfriend who was taller than him. This feeling of exhaustion became even more accentuated when A started constantly bothering them with questions about violent episodes and death, which he had learnt about from the news, in a way that was totally lacking in sentiment.

Several times during therapy I was able to discuss the themes that emerged from our first encounters with the parents. In particular I was able to help the mother not to be put off by the philosophical concerns of her son and to answer his questions in such a way as to bring him into contact with his own emotions and his own experiences of life. On more than one occasion A's father and I discussed his son's need to memorise every strategy that would be required to complete a given task, as if for him existed only the question and the answer, but not the emotional process linking the first to the second.

Some background data on V (Mrs C)

The baby was born naturally and began to suck immediately after birth. The mother recalls that early on V was *insensitive to noise and hypersensitive to touch*: a slight touch would make him jump and cry. She remembers that there was something strange about him: he had very tightly curled eyelashes and a fugitive glance, which *never focused on her*. He seemed to her to have something alien about him.

He slept little, and only at night; then towards four months he began waking up at night and staying awake for a long time. His glance was still fugitive and he started becoming *interested in noises and sounds,* an interest which soon proved to be excessive, dominating and all absorbing, capable of twisting the relationship of the child with the external world which was never looked at or touched, but only listened to. V was not, in fact, interested in objects, *he never held out his hands to take anything,* and if something was placed in the palm of his hand he would not grasp it. (*cf.* A who was like a rag doll on the bike). He made noises at the bees on the mobile above his bed, which made music, but he did not try to get hold of them. If his brother, six years older, joked and jostled him saying "boo" he would laugh like mad, but he never reached out towards his brother. He was only interested in the noise.

Weaning took place between three and six months. At eight months the baby was sent to a nursery. There was no difficulty registered at this separation from his mother. Everything apparently went well even though he already showed a tendency to isolate himself, make noises and laugh at them. During this period his maternal grandmother died of cancer and the mother went through a long period of depression.

At one year V had not started exploring, he never opened drawers or looked inside wardrobes; he only wanted objects in order to throw them down onto the floor so that they would make a noise. During this period he started sitting up. It was at this time that he was first admitted to hospital because of an unsatisfactory rate of growth. Chromosome and metabolic tests were carried out; the results were negative. At one and a half years old he was still not walking; he was admitted twice more to hospital for five or six days at a time, his mother being allowed to stay with him. The same tests were repeated (ECG CAT and metabolic tests), but the results were still negative. At two years he began saying his first words, but his behaviour was becoming more abnormal: sometimes he would look at his hands for several minutes and nothing would distract him. At three years, after a two weeks period of observation at the Children's Psychiatric Hospital he started psychotherapy following a diagnosis of psychosis.

Observations on behaviour

We will now try to describe the typical behaviour of our two patients inside the therapy room. These descriptions do not coincide with the detailed notes of one or two sessions, but are a later reconstruction of our patients' ways of being, moving and behaving which have come together after many hours of observation.

Observing A

A is a tall, clean, good looking boy, who takes pride in his appearance. He is polite and respectful. His hairstyle and clothes are simple, and very similar to the latest fashion for young people; on some occasions he reaches a high degree of social imitation, which indirectly allows me to keep up to date with the main fashion tendencies of the young. In spite of this however, those who meet him cannot help noticing that he is "different", that he is a sick boy. He is quite agile in his movements, but he is uncoordinated. His footsteps are heavy, and he is not harmonious in the way he walks; he is indecisive and full of repetitions. His speech is impetuous and somewhat mechanical. The tone of his voice is not controlled and there are no overtones in his speech so that he is unable to establish the right distance to keep from people, and he appears either too intrusive or, in spite of his loud voice, terribly far away.

A first observation: approaching the therapy room

A is always punctual for our sessions. He rings the outside doorbell in an unmistakable way, long and loudly. He comes up the stairs hurriedly, stopping suddenly once or twice on the stairway, so that he has to hold on to the handrail to regain balance and avoid falling over backwards. Other times he arrives directly behind the main door of the flat where I have my consulting rooms. In that case he knocks loudly with his fingers against the wood to get an answer and sometimes he helps the way along with gentle kicks. When he sees me he nearly always says, "Hello B," unless he gives an enormous laugh or is busy drinking Coca Cola or Sprite. He breaks off his laugh, shows me his cunning, bright eyes, stops drinking to say, "Hello B, I'm here". The impact that this greeting has on me is disconcerting: it is as if he cannot get inside me. Then A, usually lingering, moves two or three steps forwards, one or two steps backwards as if he cannot decide which way to go, and then finally goes towards the therapy room. He has heavy footsteps; he is noisy. He moves, as I am always telling him, *like a giant with his head above the clouds*. Sometimes he ignores me, and then it seems almost as if he does not recognise me; he only stops in front of the bathroom door to tell me that he has to go to the toilet. His visits to the bathroom before going into the therapy room are quite frequent.

When I make him wait in the waiting room because he has arrived too early for the appointment, he sits on the settee and begins to flip through a women's magazine in search of bare-breasted women. When it is time for him to come in, I call him but he always makes me wait a few minutes so that he can continue flipping through the magazine.

Each time his entrance takes place without a pause, he goes into the room before me: when he sees me coming he repeats, "Hello, I'm here", several times as if to tell me how clever he is. I feel as if I would like to say to him, "Who has come?" or "How much of you has been left outside?" *so strong is the sensation of being more alone than before*. He takes off his jacket, which he puts on the armchair in front of the couch. He picks it up and puts it down several times, he lays it down, he sorts it out, and then he sits or lies down on the couch.

Often, and above all on return from a break in therapy, while sitting comfortably on the couch he says, "Back at last", as if he wishes to express satisfaction and relief at being back with me again. I should feel tenderness towards him when he is like this, but in that "back at last" there is something, which freezes contact, or more precisely empties it and which is at the same time sleep inducing.

There are only two things that seem to set off some vital spark in him, which stay alive and are strong enough to capture his attention: they are my eyes and a photo of Piazza Navona taken from inside the window of a building, and which has been framed and is hanging up like a picture above the therapy couch (the photo is by Gasponi). There is probably a connection between the photo, which is mainly blue and seems to allude to an opening into some internal space, and my eyes, also blue, which he sees through the lenses of my glasses.

A second observation: inside the therapy room

The observation of how A spends his time in the therapy room, and how he moves within the space of therapy is equally interesting.

Here are some aspects:

> He is lying on his stomach on the couch as if it were a dog's basket to which he wants to become attached. His eyes are lifeless while he presses

down on his penis and kicks his feet rhythmically one against the other with his legs bent at the knees. In the meantime he makes and unmakes little piles with the coins he has brought from home, otherwise he picks up pieces of dirt, dust or threads from the carpet and rolls them between his fingers as if they were pellets. Sometimes he looks at his thumbnail, or he pushes it against another nail in order to feel a sensation of pain. He spends a long time watching the hands of his watch. Then he sticks his lips onto the cushion, as if he were kissing it or sucking it. Then, often, he goes to sleep. When he does not go to sleep, he turns over on his side, sits up again and giggles, burps, breaks wind, and sends lecherous kisses. He brings his left hand towards his mouth as if he were trying to cover up his laughter, and talks to himself in sentences full of incomplete words. His mouth is twisted, as if he were talking to a secret friend. He looks rather like a drunkard. He rubs his hands in excitement, as if to congratulate himself, he sniffs at them, he looks at me and he stops to say "Oh yes", and then he lets himself go and laughs even more riotously and emptily. In his excitement he plays with his house keys, or his moped keys, which he keeps on a long piece of string. He whirls them around in the air. He starts talking to himself again. He sends noisy kisses, rather like blowing raspberries, or lecherous kisses in the direction of my eyes. He laughs and looks at me as if he were seeking approval. His laughter too, makes me think of a drunkard. He sends more kisses one after the other. He says to himself, "The girl's shoes, or the back, the back" in a falsetto voice, violently clapping his hands and hitting his arms as if he were whipping himself.

A third observation: leaving of the therapy room

The following is a description of how A goes out of the therapy room at the end of the session. This moment is surprisingly the poorest in detail. This is because at an interactive level the session has been over for some time; sometimes it has not even begun. It is certainly the most automatic moment.

When I say that the session is over, A gets up quickly, puts on his jacket, and more or less noisily leaves the room. He says, "Bye B," without looking at me. He gives me the feeling that he wants to escape from a vague sense of unease, which forces him to think of his family, and of the journey for home he is about to set out on.

I hear him walking along the corridor tapping on all the doors he encounters with the fingers of one hand, he lightly touches the door handles. He goes out of my flat after saying goodbye to the people in the waiting room.

Observing V

V is a child with curly brown hair and large black eyes. He has a distinctive face, which is not obviously dysmorphic, but transmits a feeling of non-normality. At the outset of therapy he was very hypotonic and uncoordinated in his movements: when he walked unassisted he found it difficult to walk straight, moving forward, in a *zig-zag* manner; he did not seem to notice obstacles in his path. When he was holding his mother's hand he allowed himself to be dragged along passively without looking where he was going.

From the first period of therapy

He came to me when he was three years and four months old.

During this period he used to laugh all the time. He laughed when he was told off, when he fell over, if there was a tense atmosphere. He laughed if he heard loud noises, broke wind, or got engrossed with the poo in his bottom. Later I understood that laughing was a means of destroying and evacuating all kinds of emotions before being able to perceive them as such. If he was not allowed something, he would cry for a moment and then laugh. He could laugh in a completely uncontrolled manner, with tears in his eyes, for several minutes without stopping. He never concentrated on anything, he never looked people in the eyes, each part of his body moved independently from the rest because no attention was paid to movement, rather there seemed to be an active attempt at shifting attention away from them. He was considered hypotonic, and maybe he was, but it is certain that if we imagine attention as being a central thread connected to other threads that extend to the very limits of the body, this central thread was never properly extended and its connections with the outer threads were badly synchronised. The child often tripped over his own feet and smashed down onto the floor or against a wall. When this happened he almost never cried, he would be thrown off his balance for a few minutes (as if he were feeling either pain or fear), and then he would begin to laugh and laugh like mad. The more someone tried to stop him, the more he would laugh; above all, any change in tone of voice indicating displeasure would make him laugh all the louder. While he was laughing he would lose control of himself: he would roll on the floor, writhe and twist and sometimes hit his head against the wall. He would take off his shoes and socks and noisily clap his feet together. Often he defecated. It seemed as if he were looking for some way in which to involve me in his laughter. While he was laughing he was able to look me in the eyes strangely well and seemed to be saying, "Go on, you laugh too".

Sometimes, but more rarely, he would react by crying, but almost straight away a burst of laughter would intervene as if there were some harmful or perverse voice which deactivated the understandable answer and substituted it with its opposite.

When he spoke, the tone of his voice was very acute. He was not able to follow a conversation and answered in an automatic way to whatever was put to him. It seemed to me that echolalia was his way of blocking the entry of a question in such a way that it would not be able to provoke internal emotional echoes.

Another typical form of behaviour was that of coming up to me, sitting on my lap and cuddling me in a false way, acting like he was a new-born baby who was gurgling at his mother. This behaviour made a great impression on me: perhaps the child was mechanically repeating the emotional tones the mother had used on him earlier on and which he had registered in his memory. It was clear, however, that he repeated this on purpose each time I spoke to him about being like a baby. I felt that he was mocking me, as if he knew he was imitating what I really wanted.

Other times he would sit on my lap in a more authentic way to be cuddled or to cuddle, but the sincerity of the emotion and contact would be short lived, because he would start to laugh, and defecate or break wind.

Another typical form of behaviour during that first period was the child's tendency to enter and leave the room in such a way as to eradicate any perception of there being a difference between the waiting room and the corridor, the therapy room and the bathroom. Given that at the outset the child had no sphincter control and that the mother was trying to get him toilet trained, visits to the bathroom were very frequent. These totally prevented the therapy experience from acquiring precise boundaries. During this period V tended to evacuate every type of emotional tension through his body as if defecating represented his triumph over a foreign body which was then expelled. The therapy was, then, a continual stimulus to expel and the expulsion, followed by his exit from the room totally annulled the emotional tension and my chances of understanding and containing it. I consequently asked the mother to put him in nappies on therapy days and I no longer allowed him to leave the room. The link therapy-faeces was so evident that even the mother told me that the child, normally constipated, only defecated on therapy days, and then more than once, and then that was it for the week.

My impression was that the child, by making noises, laughing, and dirtying himself was attacking and provoking me.

Another characteristic form of behaviour inside the room was his wandering around in circles, clapping his hands or circling them like a butterfly, singing a song in total isolation and often muttering and giggling to himself. I would try tapping-knocking him on his back asking if V was there or if he had gone away. Turning round and looking at me, he would say: "Here, he is here". This sequence was transformed into a kind of game which we repeated several times during the course of therapy, and which was aimed at redirecting the child towards me if he was far away.

Remarks on observations of A and V

Both these patients seem to be struggling with the same problem: *emotions have no right of abode in their mental apparatus*. They are perceived as something foreign, which must be expelled and neutralised at any cost. It could be said that they experience emotions as "madness", an enemy to eliminate, either in full combat or by adopting bypassing tactics, or by closing themselves inside their own fortresses.

In the therapy room V soon began to manifest several different states of mind. There was *a "being a long way from me"*, as when he sang walking round in circles. In his mind he was at home or at nursery school. He repeated the teachers' words or TV jingles, all mixed up and accompanied by a bodily rhythm. Often, this "being a long way from me" became excited, full of laughter, of mutterings and accompanied by the stamping of feet, trips to the window to look at the traffic down below and the violent banging of the hands against the glass.

There was *a "being against me"*, when in an attempt at annulling my actions, he would speak over my voice, stamp his feet or hit his head against the wall, making noises or laughing violently, defecating, and wanting to go out.

Finally there were three ways of *"being with me"*: 1) a "real with me", when he would say "Here V is, he is here" and he would come up to me. 2) A "false with me", when, as I mentioned earlier he would imitate a new-born baby who through his gurgling would try to seduce the mother and 3) a "learned with me" associated with mechanical repetition of words, phrases and socially and emotionally significant behaviour which had been seen to be appreciated by me, or his parents or his teachers.

These various mental states were also recognisable in A's behaviour. When A walked with his "head above the clouds", when he was absorbed by his repetitive actions, his fetishistic excited fantasies, and his laughter, he was definitely *"a long way from the therapist"*. Instead when he looked into Dr B's eyes or at the picture by Gasponi with curiosity, he was in contact with real emotion, or with the stirrings of it; he was *"with the therapist"*. However the contact lasted only a few seconds because A would try to extinguish it almost straight away returning to his fetishistic world and to his drunken behaviour, and he would try to drag Dr B into it as well—*"against the therapist"*. On other occasions, and perhaps most frequently, A substituted false emotion for the real thing such as that expressed in his "Back at last" on his return from the holidays, or learned behaviour like the polite greetings devoid of any emotional overtones, which were sleep inducing—*"with the therapist in a false or learned way"*. In the end A would turn to sleep as a last resort in order to avoid emotional contact.

There is another important analogy in the observation of A's and V's behaviour; perhaps more than an analogy it is another key to understanding it, a point of view which summarises their behaviour in another way. These patients tend to annul any perception of there being a difference between themselves and others, they do not want to find out that the other person is not as they see him and so they try to cancel his "otherness", an "otherness" which generates emotion, either by not seeing him (distance) or by copying him (false or learned closeness, adhesiveness) or otherwise by opposing him in their typical excited way (automatic negativism), trying by every means available to involve him, seduce him or impose some degree of approval on him. *Gaining the right to exist and be seen in one's own right is extremely exhausting and at the same time a great therapeutic success.*

Fighting emotions: drunken laughter

We will return to V in order to illustrate this titanic fight against the emotions in more detail.

We had just begun making a distinction between the different mental states I outlined above when the first holidays from analysis came around. Apparently the child had not registered anything of my advance notice of the holidays: he would often laugh, it is true, but this was the norm, not the exception. This was a way of behaving that was just beginning to acquire meaning. The first day of the holidays, 24th December, the child was running a slight temperature of about thirty-eight degrees Celsius. He climbed on to the kitchen table at home laughing and "being silly" as we had decided to call it (the equivalent of the drunken behaviour of A), he fell off and began to laugh and cry until he started having convulsions; the convulsions recurred several times during the day. He was admitted to a children's psychiatric ward at the hospital where he stayed for fifteen days undergoing treatment with benzodiazepines.

Analytic therapy started up again in the normal way but fifteen days before the following interruption, for Easter, the child began crying in his sleep at night, which often woke him up. I was able to observe one of these attacks because one day the child was brought to me fast asleep and he woke up just as he was about to enter the room, crying. I took him into my arms and carried him crying into the room. There, with him still in my arms, I tried to associate the crying with the recognition of the idea of someone not being there, considering that the holidays were approaching. While I was talking, V who in the meantime had stopped crying, tried to cover up his ears and laugh (against me). Then he noticed the noise a bus was making coming from outside, so he climbed down and went to "chat" with the bus (away from me) and the sequence stopped. During the following night he had another attack of convulsions and he was admitted to hospital again. The diagnosis was secondary generalised myoclonic epilepsy, cause unknown.

During the last session before the holiday I tried to make him understand that I would not be there the next week more firmly. The child laughed like mad for most of the time, giving me very little space in which to be able to speak. After my nth attempt at talking about the holidays, he made a face as if in pain, followed by a shout of annoyance and then had another laughing fit. This sequence was repeated in exactly the same way a second time. The third time he cried a little before starting to laugh again. When I told him that the session had finished he began to sob and ran out of the room saying that he wanted his father "Go to daddy". The mother took him into the waiting room where he began to lick the radiator, while laughing and crying. It can clearly be seen from these notes how difficult it is for the child to accept emotion and hold on it without evacuating it straight away through shouting, laughing, crying, defecating or epileptic fits. Thanks only to my insistence, in the end, the emotion is able to remain inside him just enough time to allow an answer associated with it, "Going to daddy", before it is once again expelled through laughter and crying.

Normally, if I asked V: "What's your name?", he would answer echolalically, repeating the same sentence: "What's your name?" I remember one day I asked him to tell me his name, perhaps more convincingly; instead of repeating the question, he looked at me and said "V". The answer however, was followed by a furious fit of laughter during which he noisily threw all his toys on the ground, only to pick them up and throw them down again, making more noise, and laugh again. It was a real pantoclastic crisis, at the end of which he himself said: "V spoilt everything." I answered by focusing his attention on the way he refused to come near to me and listen to me; I was quite firm in trying to check his destructive behaviour. In answer to my firmness V tried crying, then laughing to make me give in, involve me, but I succeeded in containing these, by now well known tactics, within acceptable limits; so he tried to take the door stop out of the floor saying "It won't come away, it won't come away" and seemed to be pleased that it would not come away.

What the child was not able to eradicate was my firmness, a paternal quality, which prevented him from fusing and confusing himself with me as a mother, which resisted the avalanche of his faeces and his laughter let loose at the same moment in which the emotion was perceived.

A resembles V in his laughing and anally deriding the emotions that link him to his mother and his father. A careful study of his laughter, in therapy defined as the *"laughter of a drunkard"* or *"murderous laugh"* (because of its power to annihilate all emotionality), has shown that when A laughs he is thinking about an angry voice, a policeman smacking someone, the large arms of his mother which he calls *"lusmelec"* (a nonsense word), bare breasts of girls to whom he sends lecherous kisses, their pink shoes. In this way his laughter attacks the beauty of his mother (transforming aesthetic attraction into a fetishistic link), and the father's firmness, which should fix a limit to his sexual excitement. In his laughter and in his lecherous glances there is always, as with V a provocative invitation to join in with him and maybe somewhere, as V seems to show, a desire that this should not happen, (the doorstop that cannot be removed).

False and learned emotions: negative contagion

We have shown how emotions must be despoiled, destroyed or degraded at birth, and how as a result of this, internal reality remains prevalently at a bi-dimensional level, in which the objects are self-objects, dismantled, mainly sensorial, fetishistic, and totally devoid of parental function. In this situation the therapist's job beyond that of existing i.e., keeping his own three-dimensionality, diversity, and capacity for thought intact, is that of helping the patient dream his own emotion i.e., hold it within himself in such a way that it can be bound to external objects which in this way become symbolic and give origins to other symbols; to dream for the patient something which later he can dream for himself; to set off the alpha function inside him. This is a very difficult goal to reach: it seems in fact that each result obtained along the way is soon stolen by the sick part of the patient in order to prevent further progress.

As an example of this I am including some extracts from my notes on V.

> Therapy is characterised by a long period of ferocious anal attacks against my inside, with the noisy turning up-side-down of the toy box, table and chairs, all of which is accompanied by uncontrolled laughter and a great evacuation of faeces. V calls this behaviour "making a mess" and he alternates it with coming on to my lap and sucking my necklaces and pendants. When he is "making a mess" he wants me to switch the light off, and he asks me to do this in a sugary and provocative way. I think that switching off the light means switching off my eyes, my thought, my interior life with his faeces and his untidiness. I talk to him about this, and succeed in making him understand and in getting through to him emotionally. This contact, however, lasts only a short while. For months the child continues to repeat, now in a teasing way now in a boring one and always totally lacking in affection "I want to switch off the doctor" or "The light is important, it must be kept on". It seems as if the emotion felt at the beginning is quickly transformed into something learned or is expressed as a parody of the real thing and therefore falsely.

To continue on the subject of learned and false emotion I can say that for an indefinite period V continued to answer to my "What are you thinking about?" with "I am thinking about getting inside the doctor and dirtying her", as a lesson which had been learnt by heart, which he would repeat at times to please me, and others with the teasing and mocking overtones I mentioned earlier. However I am certain that at the beginning there was some contact between us on this theme. This is what I have called being with me in a false or learned way; pretending to be with me, which has made up the greater part of his way of relating to me and to the world.

Really being with me is expressed instead in a way that is never head-on, never direct. For example:

> "V makes everything a mess", shouting, laughing, breaking wind. I tell him over the noise that he wants to switch off his good mother and myself with his poo. He then stops because he feels my determination and displeasure (I am always very careful to make myself distinct from his universe of noise); he goes to the couch, he lies down and says "Mummy forgives you".

On other occasions:

> He climbs into my lap all smelly with his dirty pants, his fingers in his nose, with the falsely smiling air of someone who smarmily wants to dirty me, so I put him down and then he says to himself: "You will stay with me for ever, you will, dear little pussy!!"

One can see how he is repeating the words of a story he has been told at nursery school, or as with the first example, a phrase that his mother had said a long time before. These are profound and emotionally pertinent phrases. He is clearly upset that I am not pleased with him, but I know that he will never be able to say to me, "I want to stay with you for ever", or "I'm sorry". Direct contact is too intense for him, too scalding, so it must be weakened.

More often instead, as we observed at the beginning of this paragraph, direct contact is disconnected and substituted by false contact. Through false contact, the child gives me everything he thinks I want, except emotion. He gives me a lifeless fake emotion, as if he were giving a false "himself" as a hostage in order to escape further away, more easily. *False contacts* are typical of these patients and give rise in the counter transference to a phenomenon that we define "negative contagion": a precipitation into a world of non-thought or sleep, a switching off of the capacity to imagine. This is all the more marked, the more intense the emotion would have been had there been real contact. At the same time the therapist's emotions, if they are above a certain threshold of intensity, negatively contaminate the patient making him precipitate into a world of sleep or non-sense. Negative contagion is the result of the meeting-collision between the two totally different ways of being and of elaborating emotional data, two ways, which repel each other violently like two similar poles in a magnetic field.

The following is an extract from a session with A during his seventh year of therapy which we have included here to demonstrate at a more evolved and adult level the same slithering towards two-dimensionality that we have observed in V and the same therapeutic fight in order to keep emotion alive.

> Whilst I am about to sit down in the armchair near the therapy couch, he halts in the middle of the room, looks very closely into my eyes saying, "Hello B"; he takes some steps towards me while I am answering his greetings and comes to touch first the arm of the armchair very tenderly, and then my hand. After this contact he returns to the middle of the room, stops, and begins to grabble about in his pocket in order to take out his coins. His head now seems to be detached from his body. (He seems to have felt the contact too intense an emotion so he must detach himself, as if he is afraid to lose his identity) [...].
>
> [....] He remains uncertainly in the middle of the room. Finally he lays his jacket down on the armchair, and repeats the action once, twice, three times. His hand is clenched up in a fist. Facing me, he takes a few steps as if he were dancing, first forwards, then backwards. He adjusts his trousers several times. Finally he lies down on his tummy on the couch. Now he looks at me, his face very near to my legs, and he says "Hello B I'm fine, do you know that?" I look at him and answer that I do not believe him and I add with conviction, "What I know is that when you lie down on your tummy on the couch with a fist full of coins, you aren't OK." He answers parrot fashion, "Oh, I'm not well, you will help me won't you?" (as if he were saying things learnt by heart). To my great surprise he turns over onto his back and then sits up with his back resting on the couch, "Do you know that I talk about death?" and brings his face towards me and then moves it away

again rhythmically, starting to tell me about the deaths of various people (I understand straight away that his talking about death is an act of obedience which he makes towards his mother who had asked him to talk to me about certain things which he probably continues to talk about at home, in an obsessive and somewhat intolerable way), A begins to tell me about the death of his paternal grandfather who died when he was just over ten years old. "You know that he had breathing problems?"—and he touches his chest, miming how difficult it could be not being able to breathe.

Then after a pause, he pushes his face towards me like a wave and he tells me about his other granddad, his maternal grandfather who had "a bad heart", and he touches his heart. He repeats the same things several times, as if I were a dull child who could not understand. He does not give me a chance to open my mouth. At the same time I feel that if I go too far forward he might retreat immediately. I say to him in the end: "You seem to know a lot of things, but I don't understand what they mean to you". I ask him if he remembers anything about the first grandfather. There is a long pause, I do not know if he has understood so I repeat, "You know a lot of things, but don't you remember anything about when you stayed with the first grandfather, when he was still alive?"

After a pause he answered that he remembered that he was bald. He pauses, then, there is a torrent of things that he saw at the funeral of his second grandfather. The coffin, "I was sad", he looks at me and mimes the act of being sad, and adds: "I didn't cry because I was suffering too much." I feel that what he is telling me is a repetition of things he knows, and not things that are concerned with his real feelings. I ask him to tell me what he remembers about this second grandfather. After a pause he says with some tenderness, that he remembers when his grandfather did woodwork on the balcony of his house. Silence (it is important to make him remember his grandfather alive, keep him anchored to his experience of the grandfather). I would like to ask him other details, but A begins telling me about the murder of a girl in Rome, and of the assassinations of Falcone and Borsellino, the two Sicilian judges killed by the Mafia. He embellishes the account with details of the number of stabs in the first case, the day of the assassinations, and the age of the first judge, and repeats "Poor thing, I'm sorry", several times (he seems to reproduce the dialogues between himself and his mother for me, mixing the various elements: on the one hand I feel that there is his cold report, and on the other a mother who is trying to see sentiments and personal reactions in him and who teaches him them).

I insist on telling him that it seems to me that he wants to show me how many things he knows, but that I wonder why he has all those violent deaths on his mind. He does not follow me and I feel that my way of seeing things cannot find a place in his mind (negative contagion begins). At the nth adhesive "I'm sorry" and at a flicker of a smile which escapes him during the pause in the account, I remind him that in the past he used to let himself laugh uproariously when he thought about the death by cancer of the owner of the swimming pool he used to go to. I add that in that laughter there is perhaps, all his fears of illness. I ask him if he is afraid of illness. He says he is, very firmly and a little alarmed. I continue to point out to him that he is giggling, and I suggest that laughing about dead people is his way of keeping dead people away from him. He does not follow me. I continue to work on the possible significance of this choice of violent events, in an attempt at referring them to some internal relationship of his or some aspect of the transference, or otherwise to his image of the world. I try to tell him that perhaps he has an idea of the world being a bad and dangerous place [...]. I realise that I am imagining something that A cannot make his own, rather I feel that if I go on he will fall asleep (the tremendous experience of not being able to communicate with him, "the negative contagion"). I stop and I tell him that he knows that there are murderers and the Mafia in the world who kill people violently, and that these people are bad, so he knows he should be afraid of them. The hour has come to an end. Whilst he is putting on his jacket he says: "He has told me everything and that there is nothing more to talk about".

He is satisfied and seems calmer than usual.

The non-symbolic matrix or the triumph of the body over the mind

A and V, like many other similar children do not possess verbal, corporeal or gestural languages which contain or express emotion. Only rarely do they have the possibility of access to the symbolic and they are not able to understand the symbolic language of others. Even more serious is the fact that they seem to have a primitive, original distaste or fear of the symbolic, and appear to use their bodies in order to make sure that the mind does not develop: as soon as emotional contact is verified the body gets moving and calls attention to itself, taking it away from the moment of experience. Initially the emotion of contact is left to dwindle for lack of oxygen and then further trampled upon by bodily excitement.

We are including two more short extracts from the first therapy of A when he was eleven years old (Maiello, 1986) and from the current therapy of V (nine years old) to show how the body immediately becomes alerted, gets itself moving, in order to avoid the experience of approaching emotional contact as soon as the latter begins to impose itself on the consciousness of the patients.

> A is working on the experience of coming to therapy: he is drawing the underground which takes him to the therapist's house, and the lift that brings him up to the therapy room. He gets up and takes the dark green felt-tip. He draws many similar shapes, which to me look like the entrances and exits of tunnels [...].
>
> [...] He draws a small child next to the first tunnel, he rubs it out and draws another, bigger child who is walking. Then here is a double tunnel: he says it is dark, that it is the underground; inside the tunnels there are railway lines and a platform. He says "Barberini" (the name of the station where he gets out when he comes to therapy) [...].
>
> [...] While I am talking he makes vague scribbles on the road which goes from the station to my studio, as if it were a road leading nowhere ... then he lets himself slide down onto the floor. Touching his shoelaces he says, "Big ones don't take their shoes off" ... he touches his penis.
>
> [...] He goes back to the table and sits down again, draws a lift, then something else, which I do not understand, but which looks like a lift. Under each of these he draws something, which clearly looks like a penis. Then more vague scribbles at the bottom of the page [...]. (Maiello, 1986, p. 80)

There is a large penis which draws all of A's attention towards it, removing it from emotion; the progressive approach towards the therapy room becomes, in this way, a route without an objective which can only be learned by heart and repeated.

> V is playing with a little plastic lorry, he pushes it along the floor in circles in order to hear the noise of friction produced by the wheels against the floor (a typical game). I ask him to send me the lorry, let it come towards me, but he is not able to do so. He is able to give me the lorry, but not to push it towards me, giving up his control over its passage. I think that the lorry

> represents V who is unable to abandon himself to an emotion and who places himself either before the emotional wave or after it. Once by chance, the lorry escapes from V's hands and he then tenses himself up becoming rigid and pulling faces as if he were desperately trying to regain control both of his body and the situation, at the same time. I tell him that the lorry has come towards me and that he is not happy about it. He begins to play the same game again. In the end, when he eventually succeeds in giving up control of the lorry he looks at me and tells me that he has made a smell. I tell him that he feels his poo and smells escape from his bottom when he comes towards me […].
>
> We try to run the lorry along the floor again, and with great effort he manages to send it to me. I say "Thank you" and he answers by saying that he has made another smell. I tell him that what is happening is the same as what happened when he was little and he used to sit on my lap, but that he was not able to feel happy because straight away he had to do poo and make smells, and then he would begin to laugh; that he is full of poo and smells which escape from his bottom if he comes too close to me, and these stop him from feeling good.

This material seems to suggest that emotion is primarily felt by the child as a loss of his own bodily confines and internal contents. It is possible to hypothesise that only later are these contents, felt as exciting and potentially destructive, used against the emotion itself. There would seem to be then, an enormous excess of primitive excitement generated by emotional contact, which captures the attention of the child and is then used against his objects.

This triumph of the body over the mind is not easy to explain. We can hypothesise the predominance of a non-symbolic matrix, which crushes the symbolic matrix in analogy with what Bion (1948, [1961]) writes about regarding the basic assumptions in the life of groups. We can think of the world of minuses (-love, -hate, -knowledge), which prevent emotion from existing and developing symbolic chains. However these are only attractive descriptions, not explanations. To be truthful we do not know why emotion must be felt as being an element which is so foreign to the mind: our material suggests that there is something intolerable in its intensity, that there is something so scalding and disruptive in emotional contact that the body sets itself up as an extinguisher (this would seem to be in agreement with what Dr Meltzer (1975) says when speaking about the original mental apparatus of autistic children likening it to a nude body exposed to atmospheric agents).

What clearly happens, however, is that the experience of these people is not structured in nuclei of meaning alternated by spaces of absence. Paraphrasing one of Bion's reflections (1992): what is missing in their lives is emotional recognition both of the full spaces and the empty ones so that a beneficial turbulence giving rise and stimulus to thought is never set in motion. In therapy, the most significant moments, like approaches and separations (as we have seen) tend not to be registered as such: attention is removed from them so that they no longer represent moments of transition and discontinuity.

It is important with these patients then, to concentrate on the beginning and the end of each session, on what precedes and follows each interruption, and draw their attention to these moments of transition, in order that they are recognised in their diversity and that they are separate from the rest. At the same time it is extremely important that these patients recognise us in our diversity and otherness; that they are aware of our emotional reactions and that they learn to consider them. This is particularly important with regard to our reactions of dissent: our refusal to collude with their laughs, their false answers, and their attempts at using us as partial objects must always be clear firm and explicit. Our answers must be carefully regulated instead, on those, unfortunately rare, occasions when real emotion comes into play: joining with another in positive emotion is easily felt as a catastrophe, perhaps because, as we have mentioned earlier on, there is the inherent risk of losing confines and bodily contents. It is important to aid the survival of the emotion at least just enough to enable us to find a symbolic expression for it which may help it to remain in the patient's mind as something consistent, a knot which will later be recognised and differentiated from the empty space formed by the absence of emotion.

With these patients with such undeveloped minds who are so unemotional and who so forcefully slay emotions, it is important to keep our capacity to dream for them alive, to build symbols upon their material, giving back to it the depth and resonance from which their mental apparatus escapes. It is as if we were, at each moment, trying to blow a little soul into their bodies, to set off a spark of mental life inside them, to bring them to a really human dimension.

CHAPTER FIVE

Is it possible to interpret autistic material in the way we interpret dreams?

> Autism is a variant of thought and its development, which is based on alpha function reversal and on projective identification on the level of the part-object. By applying these two principles in an imaginative way, it could therefore be possible to interpret autistic material in the same way that we interpret dreams (Meltzer, in: Associazione Culturale Racker Venezia, 2002).

In the previous chapters on observation and the psychoanalytic method, I have shown how difficult it is, even in a specific context, such as the analytical one, to understand the behaviours of children or adolescents who suffer from pervasive developmental disorder. We saw, in my meeting with the autistic child in the ward at the Gemelli General Hospital (in the prologue), how everything that in normal personal and social relationships creates contiguity, reciprocity, arouses interest, or courtship, at first glance appears in these patients extraneous to communicative intentionality, enclosed within an unfathomable solipsism. I showed above all, with the help of Alessio's clinical data, how our difficulty in getting in contact with their way of being is not simply linked to their personal isolation, to their inability to form relations (an objective solipsism), but also to a fairly high degree of alienation from objective reality (in a pseudo-scientific manner).

It is clear at this point that the undertaking that is requested of us therapists (and at the same time of parents) is not only that of being benevolent figures, who protect the roots or the buds of their personalities from the poisons of infantile omnipotence and omniscience. The burden, both physical and mental, which we need to take into account when managing the analytic relationship, is very different from that which we experience with our neurotic and borderline psychotic patients. The processes of unconscious transference that underpin the symptoms and the inhibitions of such patients are absent or manifest themselves in a limited way, and are substituted by repetitive, idiosyncratic, excited, and flat behaviours which lack emotional meaning, and which render our efforts to reach them useless for long periods of time. In the end we observed, in the meetings with V and with A, that children and adolescents with pervasive developmental disorder, in their "being far from us", are prisoners *of feelings of omnipotence and impotence that appear to collapse into each other*. In this manner a situation develops, with its primary matrix in the body and its by-products, which prevents patients from gaining access to an awareness that a world of emotions and shared knowledge exists, in which they can participate and which they can influence in a certain manner. That which for a moment incites fear, anxiety, astonishment, surprise, instead of raising the knowledge of the Self and the Other, becomes panic, a sense of impotence and loss of boundaries, which is something unbearable and intolerable for the fragile Ego of the child; it is therefore immediately broken up, simplified and used in its concrete elements to produce automatic reactions of excitement, and manic exaltation. This makes it impossible for patients to pause for a moment on things, to take in and savour them, to keep hold of them long enough to discover their physical and functional characteristics, to organise them into recognisable structures, and to realise that these stir up emotions and sensations.

In the previous chapters I explained how our idea of development and cures has profoundly changed over the years because of the discovery, through psychoanalytic work with young and seriously ill children, of very particular phenomena of transference and counter-transference, reducible to very primitive mental processes such as projective identification with part objects (Melanie Klein), and the proto-/alpha-function (Wilfred Bion), which have proved to be the foundation of birth and the development of the child mind. I also attempted to show how these discoveries have marked profound changes in our therapeutic aptitude. In Chapter Three, "The eyes and the mind", I related it in an ideal way to the empathetic, broad and profound gaze of the mother of the premature baby, prisoner of the wires of the incubator in the intensive neonatal therapy ward, that is able to detect in the child, who clenches his fingers, not only a generic demonstration of vitality, but also a personal, "subjective" way of expressing it, as a "little rascal". Something that the distanced gaze of the neonatologist paediatrician is unable to see!

At this point some will think that I am an overly idealistic person that I am suggesting a form of understanding mental life that is hardly scientific, that I am slipping back to old dualisms and philosophical oppositions between mind and brain, between subjectivity and objectivity, between art and science. Nothing could be further from the truth. I am only saying that the experiences on which science is called to apply its capacity of discrimination and abstraction, in the study of pervasive developmental disorder, should be chiefly those arising from an active "participation" in a personal relationship with patients and not *vice versa*. In this sense it would be useful if the most recent discoveries in developmental research and neurobiology were compared with the clinical phenomena that the analytic gaze is able to detect within a therapy room. At the same time, the psychoanalytic therapist ought to fully recognise the neurophysiological context that fosters emotional development, above all in the very first stages of a child's life (Arshavsky, 2003; Robertson, 2005).

In Chapter Nine I will show how our understanding of a few clinical phenomena observed within the analytic relationship is still limited by the difficulties we have in imagining the symbolic links between primitive emotional and neurophysiological experiences.

From this point of view I have always found inspiring the studies developed by Bobath (1965) on childhood cerebral palsy, which have led to the discovery that the disorders of movements and postures in children affected by cerebral palsy are linked to the absence of normal postural and labyrinthine reflexes and their harmonious interactions. In connection with that, I would like to suggest that even in the personality development of a child with pervasive developmental disorder, when the most basic mental processes, the normal postural reflexes in my analogy, either do not switch on, or appear incorrectly, *the space left by their absence is filled by something else* that is the equivalent of spasticity in cases of childhood cerebral palsy.

At this point I would like to sharpen and test out the navigational instruments that child psychoanalysis puts at my disposal to understand the internal world of the children and the adolescents that I have in my care. I would once again like to evaluate their usefulness and effectiveness in aiding the observation and the understanding of mental phenomena, before setting out together on the journey that awaits us in the next three chapters, an adventure that is anything but easy, because it takes us through clinical landscapes that are rather uncommon.

The journey that I have chosen forms part of the initial question of this chapter, where I ask myself if it is possible—as Meltzer suggests—to interpret autistic material in the same manner as dreams: it will therefore be a journey into the clinic, similar to the interpretative exercise that one carries out when trying to attribute meaning to dreams, that, in order to be successful, involves some ability to use the concepts of projective identification and the alpha function in a creative way.

At this point, with the aim to clarify my conceptual tools in the best possible way so to allow readers who are unfamiliar with the field of my research, to begin to understand them, I quote an article written by Ornella Caccia (2012), entitled "Differences between primitive and psychotic aspects in infant mental development".

It is an article that in more scientific language expands and deepens what I wanted to express in the comparison between normal and pathological mental development in early infancy, and the development of motility in cases of cerebral palsy in children.

In her paper, Caccia explains how projective identification with part objects and the alpha-function are connatural with the *anatomy* and the *physiology* of very early life experiences, and they form the foundation of the development of the most normal primitive levels of the infant mind. It moreover shows, also through clinical examples, how these two processes can assume particular characteristics in certain circumstances, *the identification becomes intrusive and the alpha function works in reverse*, causing a stall or a modification, in a pathological or restrictive sense, of the development of primary object relations and therefore even of thinking:

> The anatomy (of the very first object relations, my addition) is made up of the characteristics of internal objects: they are part-objects, linked to a child's primitive experiences of its own body and its

> mother's (mouth, genitals, anus, faeces, surface of the skin). The experiences of the infant and the objects that attract its attention are at the beginning very fragmented precisely because of the primitiveness of its perceptive apparatus and for the transience of its attention span. In all probability, at the start it recognises that a few experiences come from a high part of its body (mouth, throat), while others feature further down (stomach, anus, genitals), a few objects press to enter within (nipple, milk), and others to exit (faeces, urine). Still in all probability, the infant classifies the first objects following criteria of sensorial and formal likeness (objects that are sticky, liquid, hard, soft, smooth or not smooth, or variously coloured). In normal development all these primitive classifications immediately incorporate an emotional quality, a sort of value judgement: objects are divided into pleasing and painful, good and bad for survival, and as such become sought after or pushed away (the primary split). Primitive objects are then joined together following a criterion of homogeneity (sensorial similarity, special contiguity, affinity and emotional correlativity). (Caccia, 2012, p. 67)
>
> [...] I believe that the healthy new-born leaves the womb equipped with a capacity for "embryonic thought" (Bion, 1959, p. 107), that is to say, the baby leaves the womb equipped with fairly well integrated and complex "preconceptions" and "proto-thoughts" of the objects that it will encounter and their functions, and it is predisposed to create links with them. Modern developmental psychology (Trevarthen, 1974; Trevarthen & Hubley, 1978; Stern, 1987), and neuroscience (Mancia, 1981) appear to be in agreement with these hypotheses. According to post-Kleinian psychoanalysis (Bion, Money-Kyrle and Meltzer) the initial preconception and the consequent first realisation is that of a breast with a nipple. (Caccia, 2012, p. 68)

Part objects for children and adolescents with pervasive developmental disorder (for example, severely psychotic patients), unlike those that have just been described in normal children, appear fragmented or badly assembled, flat and superficial, unfit to hold together the information coming from various senses or to correlate compatible emotions. They are objects that do not lend themselves to communication, that do not contribute to the discovery and to the construction of a relationship, and do not elicit that immediate empathetic recognition in the mother and in the therapist that is instead observed in the relationships with normal children:

> They are objects that refer to internal experiences that are broken up or badly assembled or dismantled (Meltzer, 1975), on which it is very difficult to build a dream, because the dream is the result of a function of abstraction of the mind that requires a certain amount of information with a minimum common denominator. (Caccia, 2012, p. 68)

One can therefore see how the characteristics of part objects, their anatomy, influence the *physiology* of the relationship of the child with itself and with the world in a positive or negative sense; they encourage or obstruct the flow of *reciprocal identification* between the child and the mother, and between the child and the therapist, that is constitutive of inter-subjectivity and human imagination:

> [...] The flow of projective identification constitutes the physiological element of the mother-child relationship through which embryonic thoughts (even labelled proto-thought or beta element) becomes an unconscious thought (the alpha element) and then a conscious thought. This is what Bion maintains when he speaks of normal or realistic projective identification and maternal day dreaming, that is to say, when he talks of physiology and not of mental development pathology. The beta element of embryonic thought is a proto-thought or proto-object (in this case it is more often defined as preconception) that is sufficiently integrated to be suitable for communication and exchange, for example, a new-born whose crying evokes an immediate empathic response in the mother. However, beta elements that are not endowed with these characteristics can exist in the infantile proto-mind, which are difficult to exchange and to consider, destined for immediate evacuation. (On this point we can think of those new-borns who immediately refuse to suckle, or who do not make eye contact, or who continually cry). These appear to be at the boundary between physiology and pathology, like tumorous cells that could recover spontaneously or degenerate and worsen into a cancer. One can think that such elements require particularly developed empathic capabilities and reverie that not all mothers are able to provide. Lastly, there exist

> beta elements that are the result of a breakdown or an attack on the maternal alpha function that begins to work in reverse, destroying rather than assigning meaning. The beta elements that are the result of this breakdown are the "bizarre objects" (Bion, 1957a, pp. 47–48) where emotional, sensorial and perceptive elements are built up in such a way that it is impossible to discover any emotional meaning. Bizarre objects are distinctly pathological or psychotic formations because not only do they not lend themselves to be thought about but also destroy the thinking process itself. (Caccia, 2012, p. 70)

There are at least two situations in which we become highly aware of the importance of conceptually keeping in mind the difference between what is "primitive" from what is "psychotic" in the anatomy and the physiology of the very first object relations.

Firstly, when we observe the behaviours of very young children in the womb or in the first months of neonatal life. In order to understand what constitutes the normal developmental processes in the transition from the physiological to the mental, we must understand which characteristics their postures, movements, and preverbal communications, such as lallation and crying, should have in order to be considered expressions of an emotional experience, and the manifestations of a personal and human mode to organise it.

Secondly, when we study the different configurations of infantile transference within psychoanalytic relation and try to understand which kind of world our patients inhabit, children or adolescents alike, and what type of experience of identity sustains their Ego. Do they live in a world of coherent and integrated part objects that are already partly meaningful or easily thinkable? Or do they live in a world of fragmented, confused, violent, incoherent part objects suitable only for evacuation and that require particular mental qualities to be understood in their emotional importance? Or do they live in a world of incomprehensibly bizarre objects that cannot be used to think?

At this point I will attempt to deepen these concepts with the help of clinical material of three patients T, S, and R, who all presented with a severe tendency of personal isolation and a failure of mental development, due in the first case, to a deficit and an immaturity in the anatomy of primitive object relations (T); in the second case, to a deficit and an immaturity of the flow of introjections and projections in the experience of identity (S); in the third case, to a state of confusion between the Self and internal objects in the structure of personality that was the consequence of a massive use of intrusive identification with part objects (R).

In this way I hope to be able to show how bodily (especially sensorial and motor) experiences and perceptions form the basis of the *grammar* of fantasy (anatomy); how the flow of identifications is the basis of *its syntax* (physiology); and the achievement of three-dimensionality in mental life the basis *of its geographical and temporal dimension* (the ability to talk about oneself).

CHAPTER SIX

Thomas (T), the child trapped in a "deaf and dumb" Pinocchio-like body: in between a disembodied mind and a dehumanised body

With the help of clinical data of Vincenzo and Antonio we saw in Chapter Four how the bodily experiences associated with an emotion do not have a right to citizenship in the mind of children and adolescents with pervasive developmental disorder, and how everything that could make them aware of an emotional experience (the observations "of sensorial impressions" as Bion would say, or the "lived body" as Maurice Merleau Ponty would say), instead of being transformed into elements apt to become dream thoughts that can then be used for thinking and for memory, is immediately dismantled, hidden, fragmented. Therefore, in the end, these patients are prisoners within a mechanical and unresponsive body, which is no longer a figment of imagination but only expression of repeated, excited or opaque "scripts", and they live in a world of bizarre, concrete, and idiosyncratic objects, not suitable for thought.

In this chapter I will talk about how motor behaviours of a child can distort and obstruct the development of its Ego and the processes of emotional and social learning, when "its actual body", its corporeality, becomes part of autistic defences and is transformed into something mute and deaf, like a piece of wood, unavailable to any commonality, unsuitable for intersubjective communication.

When I saw Thomas for the first time for a consultation, before starting a course of psychoanalytic therapy of four sessions every week for two successive years, he was five and a half years old. He was a brain-damaged child (due to anoxia at birth caused by a sudden heart attack) with a convulsive syndrome (the epileptic seizures were sufficiently controlled by medications) and presented with a serious multi-systemic delay in his development: he was still not able to stand up by himself and from the point of view of his linguistic development, he seemed to have stopped himself at the lallation stage.

Thomas has definitely been the most damaged child that I have ever been able to see within a psychotherapeutic setting, even if he is not the most serious case in an absolute sense from among all the patients I have encountered in my professional life. This put me in the position, day after day, session after session, of observing in close and direct contact his behaviour and the ways in which he interacted, and of experiencing first hand *a few peculiar vicissitudes of transference*, which had all the characteristics of a suspension of transference itself.

The request for psychotherapy

The recommendation of psychotherapy had come in the first instance from the nursery teachers who were worried by the severity of the child's personal and social isolation, which, according to them, would make it impossible to insert him into a primary school class. Thomas showed almost total rejection of every interaction with objects and people, mostly by lying on his back (notwithstanding the fact that he was able to remain seated by himself) which was accompanied by noisy kicking, staring upwards, and focusing his attention on self-stimulation. Unable to spontaneously maintain eye contact with people, on the command "look at me", he would fix his eyes on his interlocutor for a few seconds. He never used his hands for voluntary grasping. Instead he used a positive grasping within the limits of stereotypes, or he used to throw objects away from himself in a violent and automatic manner. In contrast with this, through close observation, a few of his reactions like crying, smiling, remaining silent, and nodding a few times, even if expressed in an apparently casual manner, appeared to have a meaningful link with what was done and said in that moment.

His parents had done exactly what the nursery teachers suggested in the hope that psychotherapy would help the child to break his personal and social isolation and help them to break the most exhausting aspects of their links with him.

Indeed, the mother had a strong desire to get "her own things" back. She felt trapped by her son, a prisoner within an unfulfilling relationship. She wanted to understand how to distance herself from a few of his tyrannical and irritating behaviours, like "his whining" or "his noises", without depriving him of her affection. She asked me to help her make sure that the child became more cooperative with her, and more able to fight his passive resistance that complicated even the simplest and everyday things like going to bed, sleep, food, going to the toilet, preparing to go out, and getting undressed. His father did not have much faith that therapy could help promote some change in his son's behaviour. After having consulted the best specialists in Europe, he had accepted the diagnosis that science had offered him that his son's brain was irreparably damaged. His observations of the child's behaviours were in any case considerable in their precision, richness, and detail. In some moments he described him as a small Buddha, immobile, lost in who-knows-what profound meditations, in others like a noisy war machine, continually moving, always looking for attention. He was unable to appreciate in the child, as the nursery teachers had however mentioned in their report, those small signs of opening up that revealed an albeit slight emotional involvement or participation in the external world. He admitted, however, that there was one type of behaviour in his son, which always took him by surprise and that filled him with tenderness. Every time that he sat on the sofa at home, Thomas immediately approached him, shuffling forward on his bottom and stretched himself out perpendicularly to his body with his neck resting on his knees.

Clinical data

The observations of the parents and of the staff of educational and medical services (nursery teachers and doctors) on the modality of T's being in the world and his interpersonal relations made me immediately get an idea of what kind of child I would meet. Even before seeing him in the consulting room, I thought that, like all the other people who had known T for a long time, I would have to face the inertia of his illness, the impact of his omnipotent control on reality, and the dramatic consequences, at an emotional level—in my internal experience—of the simplification and repetitive nature of his behaviours. I expected that my normal navigational instruments would show their inadequacy above all in helping me to contrast the danger of being dragged into a personal relationship, which was saturated with signals, and into a stereotypical intercourse of questions and answers lacking in emotional meaning.

The first assessment meeting

When I met him for the first time T was leaning against his mother's body with his head turned back behind her left shoulder. He was awake but completely detached from all he was experiencing, except, perhaps, hearing. He kept his arms straight along his body. When his mother started to separate from him and hand him over to me, almost imperceptibly T tried to cling even more to her breast and shoulder, but he did not resist being transferred to my arms. He did not use his hands to hold on to her, to keep her close to him, or to reject me, and he did not cry. He did not look me in the eye when I called him by name, in an attempt to get his attention. He refused to lean on my chest while I supported his back. Instead, he sat up on my hand and started to move his little hands and arms in an uncoordinated manner, as if he were drowning, realising that he could not hold on to anything solid.

Instinctively, I grabbed his hands and held them firmly inside the palm of my right hand, intending to give him the feeling of being held. This seemed to calm him down a little, but it did not make any change in terms of attracting his attention, so I told him that he was certainly frightened to be in the arms of a doctor whom he did not know, and for this reason he was trying to distance himself from me by arching back and putting his hands in between us to keep me away.

Once in the playroom, I sat him on my lap, with his face raised towards the window overlooking the garden. If T had earlier used his hands to keep me at a distance, now that he was sitting on my lap he rejected to lean against my chest. Instead, he started struggling with his head, moving it rhythmically from side to side, and he even attempted to bite my hand. For this reason I placed him on the couch and I sat next to him.

I immediately noticed how easy it was for him to sit up straight all by himself. I was also struck by the fact that he never used his hands to support himself on the sides or to turn around or change his position and lie down. He did not show any sign of spasticity. On one occasion, maybe by chance, he slid on one side and found himself in a prone position. For a moment he started crawling and turned his eyes wide open towards me, but without seeing me. Immediately after that, as if feeling irresistibly heavy, he collapsed into himself. He lay on the couch face down for a few seconds, motionless like a "little dead body". Then, without any help from me, he lay face up and started to bang his feet frantically against the wall; he banged his right foot against his left leg; he grabbed his left toe with his hand (he was not wearing shoes), and he tried to move his left foot towards his face. He became "a noisy war machine", as his father had described him. With all this noise he seemed to want his mother to hear him from the waiting room, to send out a strong call for help. As a matter of fact, he alternated motor activity with brief pauses of silence, during which he seemed to be in a listening attitude. Then he started to slide on his back until, without looking at me, he was able to make a ninety-degree turn and rest his head on my lap, as if it were a cushion. At this point he calmed down and remained motionless for a few minutes, looking at the light from the window. He did not seem to acknowledge my body at all, or me as a person. For a long time he ignored my hand, which I had discreetly placed on his chest, to make him feel my presence. His eyes were "opaque", devoid of light, completely turned inwards. I did not understand whether he was sad, disappointed, angry or simply estranged.

An imperative: to cancel otherness

In these notes about the initial moments of the first assessment meeting, we can see how T copes with the separation from his mother and the experience of meeting, for the first time, a new person, unknown to him, in an unfamiliar place. What is immediately striking is that the child, despite the absence of abnormal muscular tone, postures and movements, deficits in grasping or visual impairments, never uses his hands or his eyes in order to regulate his proximity or distance from people.

When he is about to be placed into my arms, he makes no attempt to hold on to his mother; he does not grab her blouse, does not stare at her with greater intensity and does not cry desperately. He only sends out an imperceptible signal, showing that he wants to oppose his new situation, by abandoning himself even more passively on her shoulders like "a sack of potatoes".

When he is suspended in mid-air he does not use his eyes or hands to reject me. He refuses to look at me when I ask him to do so and call him by name. Instead, he starts moving his hands and arms in the air aimlessly and violently, like a blind child. His flapping occupies the space that separates our faces. He does not convey anxiety, but only a vague sense of pain. He is so lost in his gestures that he cancels any perception of reality. His movements resemble the uncoordinated and fragmented involuntary gestures or tremors of neonates, when they are moved from one breast to the other, or when they are placed in their cot because of their physiological immaturity or because they are not sufficiently held or well oriented due to their mother's inability to hold them.

Later, one can notice that when I try to draw his attention on me by squeezing his hands in my right hand and offering a secure support for his back and bottom with my left hand, so that he is well seated, straight in the middle, facing me, T rebels and starts struggling, throwing himself about, showing his active rejection due to anxiety. A moment later, he makes the same movements when he sits on my lap. When I invite him with a gentle push of my hand to lie on my chest, he reacts by biting it.

What is most striking, however, is the speed with which the child is able to transform the novelty of our encounter in something known and familiar, following in the session the same old scripts of what he does at home: the noisy "war machine" sounds and the quiet moments on his father's lap.

These "scripts" seem to contain an embryonic capacity to retrieve his absent object, like in those brief pauses of silence when he seems to stay in a holding position. These are like small inserts, intervals or crevices with which he uses to check whether his object has heard his calls. Fleeting moments of opening up that are soon replaced with chaotic and noisy movements.

To this regard, it is interesting to notice that in both situations the child lies on his back, as if a hard surface under his head and back helped him feel more self-confident; as if that position helped him to feel again, or to recover the memory of his back touching the hard walls of the uterus, or as if he felt he could give more strength and vitality to his noisy movements. He never spontaneously chooses to lie face down. We know that, at home, he refuses to walk on all fours and he prefers to move across the floor shuffling his bottom. However, the moment when, by chance, he finds himself on all fours, to my great surprise he opens his eyes almost automatically, even if he does not seem to see anything.

> […] After a while T started banging noisily his legs and feet against the couch and the walls of the therapy room. In addition to that, inhaling and exhaling in a rather uncoordinated manner, he began making raspy sounds with his saliva, drooling on the sides of his mouth. These unpleasant sounds alternated with a series of melodious "ma-ma" and "pa-pa", which he tended to keep in his throat lacking the strength of a proper call for help. This melody seemed to get lost into the void like a solitary song that does not receive a reply.
>
> Then these sounds disappeared completely and in a crescendo of noisy excitement the child began to rhythmically touch his lips with his left hand as if he wanted to break the sounds or his breathe. He also tried to put his right thumb into his mouth. At first, he was unsuccessful because his moving tongue occupied all the space in his mouth and pushed it out. Then finally, he was able to lodge it between his gums and the inner part of his cheek. As he sucked his finger this way, he began to repeatedly bang his right hand (with the thumb in his mouth) against his left hand. At a certain point, without warning and without looking at me, he grabbed my thumb (my hand was still resting on his chest). He moved it closer to his mouth and started banging it instead of using his own hand. On several occasions in the course of this session, he alternated an orgy of movements and noises of his mouth and his limbs with moments of absolute immobility during which he was struggling with an undefined unease, a sort of nausea […] at a certain point, the loud noise of an accelerating motorcycle on the slope near my office seemed to get inside him like a violent wave. Then the child became motionless, overwhelmed by a painful and incomprehensible experience. He became completely absorbed, listening to something that was happening within himself. In the end, he farted and maybe also defecated a little in his nappy […].

The confusion between internal and external

The clinical material of this part of our meeting is particularly interesting because it shows how limited and fragile the differentiation between internal and external is in the child's relationship with reality; how the internal world tends to be easily confused with the external world and *vice versa;* and how all this hinders the child's confidence of being able to transform external reality.

Let us observe first of all how each noise gets into him from outside without encountering any obstacle and causes an undefined unease, a physical discomfort, like nausea, that captures completely his attention: participating to this experience caused me great pain and alarm. His ability to filter painful or intense stimuli coming from inside or outside his body is scarce. He is easily overwhelmed. In these situations, his eyes become glazed, as if covered by a transparent veil, or his general posture resembles "a little dead body" due to a momentary suspension of spontaneous movement. Another striking aspect of our encounter is the child's deep conflict between wishing to draw the object closer to him and giving it up, between surrendering to the object and managing everything by himself. The strength of his melodious "ma-ma" and "pa-pa" sounds are feeble and their music seems to get lost in the wind, into nothingness, as if the child himself could not believe in the existence of an object ready to welcome and amplify them. Verbal language, just like his hands, does not establish a link: the child does not use either to look for the object or to attract it to himself. The melodious call of his vocalisations is soon replaced by the noises of the orgy of his movements and his raspy, throaty sounds.

Finally, we can observe that in this part of our meeting, the actions of the child focus on his mouth and the relationship between what is inside it and what is moved near or inside it from the outside. It is not easy to understand the meaning of this activity, during which he interrupts the other movements of his body. There is a great production of saliva, many unpleasant raspy sounds and there is a turgid, ever moving tongue which occupies his throat and mouth: in brief, there is a host of internal characters who struggle to interact with other characters from the outside, like the hands and fingers that he moves closer to his lips, wanting to get in. This noisy and meaningless performance, on the stage of "the theatre of the mouth" is once again used by the child to create an omnipotent feeling of great self-sufficiency, which does not allow him to build a representation, albeit primitive, of the world. Observing him, I also had the impression that his wish to suck his thumb was not only hindered from within, by his tongue, but also by the expectation of an external prohibition. There is one hand hitting another, something like a harsh and punitive Superego, when it moves closer to his lips.

> [...] Towards the end of the session, in an apparently fortuitous manner, while he was sitting on my lap, T fixed his gaze on me and stopped ignoring me for a moment. He looked me in the eye for a long time and then,

suddenly, he burst out crying desperately, as if a sharp arrow has pierced his forehead, causing him excruciating physical pain. For a moment, I thought of an anxiety attack, linked to the fact that the child had suddenly realised that I was a person different from his mother or another familiar figure. I talked to him about this, but I didn't manage to calm him down. Then I placed him on my shoulder. I immediately realised that the word "ma-ma", which I had used in my interpretation, did not evoke in him any emotion or memory, which could connect him to the real mother who was waiting for him outside. So, I talked to him about my eyes, of how he experiences them as bad and dangerous, like two hard and penetrating nipples. T stopped crying desperately and began whimpering; he went on like that for almost the rest of the session, until he fell asleep, exhausted. This was the only moment in which I was able to notice and active use of his eyes. For the rest of the time, he moved them along the walls of the room or gazed at the light from the window, giving me the impression that he was able to see everything around him but was unable to take in what he saw and keep a personal memory of his encounter with me and with the play room, as if he suffered from some kind of "constructive apraxia", a sort of inability to grasp the whole context, landscape, stage, theatre, geography of the place where he is, even before being able to discover its single structural or functional elements, including also depth.

Gradually opening up to reality

In a general framework of control, therefore, there are some exceptional moments in which the child shows his ability to spontaneously leave his isolation and motor stereotypies. However, considering the consequences of his opening up, one immediately understands how painful it is for him to give up his pathological defences.

As the nursery teachers and the physiatrist who had already assessed the child's psycho-motor development—had pointed out, the clinical material of this initial meeting shows that T's behaviours cannot be interpreted simply as an expression and a consequence of his original neurologic lesions and mental delay. This, indeed, gives strength to the idea that his psycho-motor delay is due, at least in part, to his refusal to unlock his full potential. The impression is that a secondary deficit in his development, linked to personality and relational disorders, has come into being. The child's cognitive and mental delay seems to be made even more serious by his refusal to expand his perceptual and emotional experience beyond a small number of very limited and repetitive motor and attachment behaviours.

At the same time, if one looks at his current symptoms and attempts to reconstruct his past, one wonders in which way some specific experiences in the early months of neonatal life may have influenced his birth to psychic life. It might be interesting to investigate how his early pathological sensorial and motor experiences (muscular tone, posture, motility, irritability and impotence, epilepsy) may have affected the quality of his primary relationships, and what obstacles, delays, and distortions they may have produced in the development of symbolic processes, among which verbal language. In particular, it could be very interesting to investigate how the difficulties that the child experienced in his early months of life when trying to grasp objects with his hands, might have negatively affected his feeling of being an active subject in the transformation and possession of reality.

In this sense, the complete reading of the notes of the third consultation meeting may be quite evocative.

The third consultation meeting

T arrives held in his mother's arms. His head sticks out beyond her shoulder His arms are dangling along his body. As soon as he sees me, as I say hello to him and call him by his name, he smiles faintly and adheres to his mother's body even more. He does not use his hands to hold on to her, however, and lets her put him in my arms without resistance. He rests on my chest, with his head on my shoulders, like a bag of potatoes. He does not cry and does not look at his mother as she goes to the waiting room. In the children's room, without any resistance, he lets me seat him on the couch next to the toy-box, while I sit next to him. I notice that he looks at me more than once, smiling, alternating his eyes on me with protracted looks (or lingering glances) towards the light behind my head: a white, round lamp hanging from the ceiling.

He looks less persecuted today, less "opaque". He pays attention to the world around him. He smiles as if he wanted to screen himself and be looked for. However, the way he looks at things seem of little depth: it is as if his eyes "caressed" the surface of things or were "blinded" by lights, without being able to take in the space, background and depth of things.

While he is busy looking around, in an apparently casual manner he grabs the basket of toys, shakes it and dumps it on the couch. He takes a hard, transparent plastic bag containing some families of farm and wild animals, shakes it without looking at it until he empties it, and then he starts playing with it using his hands, in a crescendo of frenzied and noisy excitement. At first he sits, but then he lies down, still holding the bag firmly with one hand and using the other to hit it or to pull it in another direction. He rubs it against his face and eyes, and then he places it on his lips and mouth for a while. The excitement in his hands and arms is accompanied by the constant agitation of his legs and feet, which he violently bangs against the mattress or the walls. At the same time, he mumbles, inhales or exhales continuously, pausing from time to time. In order to try to calm him down, on one occasion, I rest my hand on his chest. My watch makes him curious, and he pauses for a while to look at it, maybe because of its brightness, stopping making noise.

I am struck by the way he plays with the plastic bag with his hands; it almost looks like the representation of a situation of conflict between the will of the child and that of his parents. When he holds it tight with his right hand, there comes the left hand, apparently trying to interrupt this exclusive possession in a nasty manner: it strikes the other hand, as if to say "drop the bag", or it tries to take it away, as if trying to overcome the stubborn habit of putting something dirty or dangerous into his mouth. I talk to him directly, expressing my thoughts about this to him, and as I speak I notice, to my great surprise, that the child is listening to me, silent and motionless. The end of the session is approaching, and I remind him a few times. At the same time, I ask him to give me the plastic bag so that I can put in it all the toy animals that are scattered on the couch and on the floor. T does not listen to me and starts making his noisy rituals once again. At the end of the hour, very gently and looking him in the eye, I take the plastic bag from him, without asking for his permission. Strangely, T does not protest, also because I distract him, as I hold the little plastic bag in full sight in front of his eyes. As I slowly fill it up with the toy animals, naming them one by one, I use my eyes to guide his eyes on my movements. He is interested in this scene, and he does not stop looking. He seems particularly fascinated by the fact that all the toys get into a container and are kept in there. Finally, I orderly put it back in the toy box. As I by now feel ready to take T to his mother, to my great surprise he grabs my hand and with it he plays the same game as he did before with the plastic bag. Then he lets it go and repeats the same game, this time using one if his little hands. Our time is up now, and I pick him up and rest him on my shoulder. Before leaving, I let him "say good-bye to the room", turning around 360 degrees. Outside the room, I notice

that the child looks absent and lost, no longer able to pay attention to me, or to return my final goodbye.

The phenomenon of transference suspension

The clinical picture that emerges from these notes appears rather contradictory and complex. T's behaviours, which initially seem similar to those of a much younger child, maybe just a few months old, tend to repeat themselves forever, unlike in normal development, and their automatism destroy any expectation for change. It is difficult to see a future inside any of them. They might be compared to the flapping of wings of penguins, which never turns into flight, where the *frequency of the gesture only produces meaningless din*. T is a child who uses his objects (the plastic bag), parts of his body (and mine), and also some of his internal contents to produce repetitive sounds and noises. His "noisy war machine" behaviours (noisily rubbing or hitting with his limbs, the raspy sound of saliva in his throat)—*which are, somehow, quite likely to preserve the meaning of calling his object to himself*—take on an orgiastic connotation that absorbs his attention completely, altogether distancing him from reality, from the awareness of his own Self and the Other, from his body and that of anyone close to him. The child then becomes emotionally inaccessible, "deaf" to any suggestion to move towards greater motor or linguistic autonomy. His powerful and lively actions are confused with the search for frenzied excitement, as if he wanted to show to himself that he is strong and lively on the basis of the identification with what makes him most anxious (noises), in a sort of endless, step by step progression, because what frightens him keeps reappearing, in the form of nameless dread.

Moreover, there are other moments when there is a suspension of attention (and consequently also of the transference experience), when the child is completely absorbed by "painful" physical sensations, which are triggered by the incursion of an intense sensorial stimulus from the outside into his body. All that is needed is the gusting sound of motorcycle revving, the barking of a dog, the ringing of a mobile phone, or the crying of a child to activate his intestinal peristalsis, with the appearance of colic pains, nausea, stinks, and poos over which he seems to have no control and by which he feels persecuted. In such moments, T gives the impression of being easily dragged away in a "passive" way, like in the rapids of a river, of being overwhelmed by something intolerable, like a storm of unpleasant physical sensations (nausea), which he can do nothing about but suffer. He keeps his eyes open, but he does not seem to see what is around him; he is like a blind, silent child, motionless like a "little dead body", or a little Buddha. *Maybe in this way he pretends to make himself invisible so as to magically annihilate his persecutor.*

The moment when he is able to get out of this situation, or he is somehow expelled from it, T is unable—or unwilling—to actively use his hands to hold on to his object: he "spreads himself" on his mother's body, *as if he had no notion of a nipple*; the same applies to his eyes, which seem to "slide" over things and people, and fix on bright objects, like those of a much younger child. He seldom manages to use the eyes of the Other to get inside his or her head as if he had no notion of an object with an internal space provided with *ports of entry*: people's eyes do not seem to be perceived by him as objects that invite him to enter into a three-dimensional space. What is the deep reason for this psychological disaster, I ask myself. There is, perhaps, something very "painful" in the awareness of his dependence, but also of his being "alone", and therefore that part of his psychic apparatus that might allow him to work through such an experience is immediately dismantled!

What can be observed on the whole, then, is only a series of excited states without the presence of emotions but only of physical sensations that leave no space for any affective communication, and moments of "opacity" or blockage, in which a painful experience is so intense and mysterious that it completely overwhelms the fragile Ego of the child. There is also a certain circularity between these different states, so that excitement seems to be the child's way of avoid the "heaviness" of opacity or blockage, or it may become the element that triggers his painful experience of blockage. What is most remarkable in his behaviour is—to use a geometric model—the repetitiveness of his actions has a circular pattern, which never becomes a spiral. His sensorial experience seems incapable of reaching the threshold of emotion and of promoting the birth of a mental thinking apparatus.

At this point one might wonder how the therapist can help the child to get out of these meaningless states. How can the therapist mentally survive the excitement and the opacity of the child?

The initial answer could be of a muscular type: one must find a way to gaze somehow, forcing him to open up. The risk is that one might kill the flower by "shaking its bud". In fact, before acting, one perhaps needs to analyse the clinical material more accurately, in order to understand if and when the child spontaneously goes back to the transference.

As I have noticed before, there are moments when T seems to be a younger, more active child, who actively takes part in the relationship, even if at a part-object level. *There is something in his behaviours that, albeit primitive, fleeting and transient, belongs to development*. He is able, even if quite rarely, to use his gaze to latch on to my eyes, or the smile in his eyes to call me close to him. At the same time, the clinical material shows that this experience of contact quickly turns into something persecutory, which causes a painful obstruction in his forehead, or continues to be superficial and two-dimensional. He grabs my hand and takes one of my fingers to his mouth, even if something prevents him from sucking or biting it. He seems to be aware that there are surfaces on the bodies of adults on which one can rest, or postures that establish a relationship between his body and mine, that reassures him. Moreover, in the silence, which is present in the room the moment when he suspends his noisy activities, he seems to "actively" start waiting for someone or something to enter into his experiential field once again. His behaviour makes me think of the approaching of voices or steps that remind him of known presences, like his mother or some other relative. These are situations in which the waiting for, and the realisation of a very concrete interpersonal relationship take shape—even if they do not last long—are almost immediately replaced by his stereotyped and controlling behaviours.

Along with his one- and two-dimensional polarities, therefore, there are rare moments in which he moves towards a three-dimensional reality. As we have noticed, he allows himself to be *"wrapped by silence"* for a few minutes (when he stops making noises and waits to hear his mother's steps); or to be *"wrapped by the light in the eyes of the Other"*; or *"by the voice or words of the Other"* (when he utters sweet, musical syllables that sound like little speeches, or when he smiles blissfully to himself, as if he were thinking about something pleasant). In such moments one has tender feelings about T because in his behaviour one can finally perceive a search for the absent object and an appreciation of the present object.

However, we can also see how these invitations are fleeting and transient, how silence is perceived soon as dangerous and painful, how his way of looking at things is superficial, and how he latches on to familiar surfaces, in search for safety. At the same time we observe the presence of two clinical phenomena: together with the weakness of his calling, there is a certain degree of sliding, a spreading of himself on things. The consequence of it is the fact that the less intense the calling is, the more his adhesiveness becomes solitude, distance, and sensory self-stimulation, thus losing every emotional and communicative connotation.

We then discover that such tendencies, which reveal something primitive in the child's way of being, do not foster development because of the substantial inadequacy of the child's internal and external objects to get to know them, understand them, stabilise them and reinforce them (*like letting a child suffering from cerebral palsy evolve without therapy*).

Unfortunately, the incompleteness of my notes does not allow me to faithfully reconstruct the evolution of infantile transference within T's therapeutic process in the two years that followed the initial consultation sessions, and consequently I am unable to give the reader the possibility of following its transformations step by step. I can only say that the child learned to become more interested in reality, to be more cooperative with the people around him, only when I managed to make him experience a tolerable level of anxiety and depression within his relationship with me. I started to stop responding in an automatic manner to his requests for safety and control, and being subjected to his negativistic behaviours. At the same time, I offered him a mental and physical contact that was more appropriate and respectful of his non-integrated and disintegrated mental states, particularly at the beginning and the end of our sessions, and during the separations and interruptions of therapy. Thus, I was able to keep him well oriented, for longer periods, at a deeply emotional level, in space and time, towards his objects of dependence, his mother in particular.

What follows is the transcription of two initial and two final sessions that clearly illustrate this type of therapeutic interaction.

The economy of anxiety: from omnipotent control to green light, first access permissions

Thomas (at the beginning of therapy)

T arrives in his mother's arms like a sack of potatoes, with his head leaning out beyond her shoulders. He doesn't look at me, even if I repeatedly greet him calling him by name; he remains passive, leaning on his mother's body, until I pick him up in my arms. I notice that as soon as I get closer to his mother, he starts to rhythmically rattle his teeth [...] at this point, in the silent room, one can only hear the ticking of his teeth. "Tic tic tic". Holding him in my arms with his head on my left shoulder, I take him to the playroom. I close the door and I place him on the couch sitting up. I sit next to him so that he can see me, but he ignores me. He immediately lies down on the couch and turns until he can place himself perpendicularly to me and rest his head on my knees. He keeps rattling his teeth. I imitate the noise of his teeth, trying to identify myself with him or to arouse in him some interested about me, but to no avail. He keeps rattling his teeth, completely absorbed in this activity. At a certain point I tell him that he sounds like a mechanical doll and I ask him what happened to T the child. He starts staring at the lamp lit in the middle of the ceiling and he stops rattling his teeth for a while, but then, still staring at the lamp, he starts doing it again. I remark that he is looking at the lamp, which is full of light and warmth as if it were his mother's breasts, while he rattles his teeth like a baby who is very cold and afraid. He looks at my chest. I repeat my comment adding that beside the warm breast-lamp outside him, perhaps he feels he has a bad and cold breast inside him. I don't know how much he understands my interpretation, but I notice that the more I talk to him and the more convinced I sound, the more he calms down and manages to focus his attention on the lamp. At a certain point, he stops rattling his teeth and starts mumbling in a repeated sequence of throat sounds, with ample movement of his tongue and large production of saliva; his initial "joy" is immediately replaced by a strange excitement that gradually spreads to his arms and one of his legs which he starts banging on the couch. The feeling that he conveys is that of a child who wants to hide but at the same time wants to be caught and noticed. He suddenly stops, looking tired. He tries to stick his right thumb in his mouth to suck it, but he cannot because his tongue keeps moving as he mumbles. His thumb then slides under his gums until his tongue stops and then it can finally find its space in his mouth. He starts sucking it: I comment that his thumb struggled to find a place where to be sucked, because of his restless mouth and I add that also my words seem not to find a space inside him, as if they were dangerous and hard. After a few moments of calm and silent sucking, he takes his thumb out of his mouth and once again starts rattling his teeth and moving his arms and legs frantically, as if all his energy had come back. I tell him that perhaps he is telling me about his fears when he is in his little bed at night and of his ways of making himself heard by mummy and daddy so that they come and take him to their big bed, between them. He stops moving and his mouth is closed. Is he afraid of being punished perhaps? In truth, I am not sure that he is "listening to me"; rather, he seems to be following his own script, an old recording whose words I cannot grasp. A moment later, he starts making several farts, poos in his nappy and blows a couple of raspberries with his mouth, followed by an open-mouthed loud laughter of real satisfaction. I talk to him about his pleasure in making noises with his bottom and his mouth and of his satisfaction in feeling a powerful stinker (he understands this) in my room, but I also talk about his fear that I might get angry about his wish to bombard me and soil me with poo and stinks, as well as the other children who come to my playroom. I tell him that he is afraid that I might become a harsh, bad, punishing daddy. Another moment of tiredness follows. He settles on my knees and remains calm for a few minutes. I start talking to him about the end of the session. Apparently, he seems not to understand or to ignore what I am talking about, he starts rattling his teeth again, becoming more and more distant and "opaque". I tell him that we'll go back to his mummy soon, but the fact that I talk to him about his mother does not to seem arouse any emotional reaction in him: he is lost in his opacity. I ask him to tell me if he wants me to pick him up and take him to his mother, or if he wants to leave the room on his own feet, but he behaves as if he didn't hear me. So I make him stand up putting him in front of me. I notice that he is able to stand up by himself, holding on with his hands on my arms, but I feel that I am forcing him to do something, which has no meaning for him at all. In him, I notice a sort of total passivity and lack of attention for what is happening, just like at the beginning of the session, moving from his mother's shoulders to mine. So I pick him up holding him so that he can look around. I take a little walk up and down the room, left and right, saying goodbye to everything I see, reminding him that the room will be waiting for him until tomorrow, but T remains completely uninvolved in this ritual. He seems absorbed by something inside him. He has switched off all the lights within him. When he leaves, resting on his mother's shoulder, he doesn't look at me, as I say goodbye, apparently not even able to hear my voice.

Thomas (five years and nine months)

T arrives in his mother's arms slumped on her shoulder. As they cross the threshold, he slightly bangs his head against the doorjamb and starts whining. The mother doesn't seem to notice this little incident and instead she shows me a little hematoma under the child's chin due to an accidental fall the day before. In the passage from his mother's arms to mine, T keeps being passive. As we go towards the playroom, I notice how lost he looks, as if he did not remember anything about this place or didn't have the strength or the will to be interested in it. For this reason, instead of placing him immediately on the couch as in our previous sessions, I keep him on my knees. To my great surprise, the child suddenly lights up and shows me that he wants to take his favourite position, which is lying on the couch perpendicular to me, resting his head on my knees, just as he does with his father when they are together on the sofa. Once he lies down, he starts playing with his hands and mouth in a very excited way. Today, his play consists in "breaking" the air and the sounds from his mouth, banging one hand on his lips, alternating this activity with the usual excited movements of his arms and legs. He avoids looking at me, even if sometimes he quickly glances at me without pausing and without showing any sign of recognition. He often sits up and then the sound and the power of his excited play increase in intensity. Then, he puts his head on my knees again and remains motionless, staring in front of him in a state of suspension. I feel like a prisoner of an experience that does not belong to me and that annihilates my presence. Thus, I decide to escape from his omnipotent control and for the first time, very gently, I remove my legs from under his head, replacing them with a soft cushion and I sit on the couch opposite his feet. Then T, with all his strength, tries to turn around and take his previous position, but without success, because I don't let him do it, moving away from the couch and sitting on a chair close to him. At this point, as I talk to him, saying that he cannot stand the fact that I am free to move as I like and telling him that I am not his daddy, and that this room is not his home, he shows me all his repertoire of noisy, stereotyped movements with his arms and legs and his oral stimulations, sticking all his right thumb and stimulating the inside of his cheek. At a certain point, a few minutes after these demonstrations of self-sufficiency and arrogance, I feel that all this excitement is overwhelming him: so I take his hand, I hold it tight and I place it on his chest to make him understand that I am there and that I want to hold him, clearly in my own way. Feeling this contact, T reacts letting me know that he wants to be helped to sit up and then to stand. Once standing in front of me, however, he cannot even take one step, either forward or backward, so I place him on my knees again holding him towards my face. At this point, he starts alternating movements: he comes closer to me to gently grab my hair while his other hand strikes my head and then he throws himself backwards arching his back. I tell him that he wants to get into my head knocking (I mimic the knock-knock sound and he laughs) but perhaps he thinks that there is someone behind him that forbids him to do it, and so he must stop knocking and check. I also notice that as he plays with the upper part of my face, he completely ignores my eyes and glasses, behaving as if they don't exist, and he seems unable to think of the eyes as the natural portal to get into the internal world of a person. The session is now almost over and I put him back on the couch. Mindful of what happened in the previous session, I tell him in advance that we will soon go back to his mummy who is waiting for him in the room outside. He starts whining and complaining, but I do not understand this cry and I do not immediately respond to it. I move my chair closer to the couch where he is now lying and I move his body to make sure that he is comfortable and that there are no physical problems, thus reducing the distance between us. For a while, I hold his hands in mine and when I feel that he begins to resist my hold, I let him free and I rest my hand on his chest, sitting so that he can easily meet my eyes. As soon as I let him go, T grabs the blanket and covers himself up including his face, sucking his hand greedily. Then he stops sucking and with the same hand he grabs mine, taking it to his mouth, but his other hand immediately intervenes, hitting it, and his whining resumes. I try to understand if he wishes to go back to his mummy and I tell him about it. As I mention her, I have the feeling that he does not remember his mother and that he cannot find her image inside him. It is now time to go: I stand up and I pick him up in my arms, I start walking around the room, naming all the objects that I see and I make him say goodbye to them. To my great surprise, I notice that his gaze is different this time: he seems to be seeing the room for the first time. This gives me the indirect proof that resisting his immediate requests for protection, offering him a different way of being near him without automatically wrapping him up like in a blanket or not allowing him to slump on my body when he is troubled or distressed drives him to "open his eyes" to external reality. I take him back to the waiting room. The mother seems surprised to see us. As I hand the child to her, I ask her not to put on her sunglasses straight away and not to be in a hurry to leave. I invite her to pause a moment and to help her child find her again, even if T has annoyingly started whining once again.

Living beyond excitement and opacity: a new awareness

Resisting without violence or rigidity his attempts to slump on my knees, or his expectations to be immediately picked up when he starts whining, letting him cry a little without comforting him at once: all this seems to lead T to take new initiatives, like exploring space and looking at reality with "eyes wide open". Reducing the immediate and automatic protective response of a physical and sensorial contact seems to allow him to transform himself from a "doll-bag of potatoes" into a "true, lively, exploring child". All this should not make us feel easily enthusiastic, because we can also see how renouncing the protective "blanket" in which he is wrapped by his mother or in which he actively hides like on his father's lap, makes T face new experiences of reality that can arouse his interest but can also easily become persecutory and confused because *they put him in touch with the serious limitations of his development*. We can also notice that his relationship with me is still mainly instrumental, even if I am quite relieved when I see that the child, on certain conditions, is available to more complex motor experiences, like wanting to be propped in order to stand up and try walking and to new stimulations from the objects in the therapy room. It is interesting to observe what happens in moments when patients with a pervasive developmental disorder like T abandon their fantasies of omnipotence and impotence and make themselves available to a contact with reality. It is a very painful moment, particularly for the people who are around them and love them, because one becomes aware of how these patients are disarmed *vis-à-vis* reality. Opening his eyes to reality is exciting and stimulating for T, but it is also dangerous; it is like finding oneself in a condition of powerfulness/powerlessness, very similar to the one experienced as babies. The new things that he finally grabs with his eyes or with his other senses, whether they are objects, spaces in the room, my eyes or my hand, catch his attention for a moment but do not seem to find a natural support in his imagination or his capacities: he reacts as if he didn't know what to do and he behaves as if all this made no sense to him; he still does not seem ready to find his bearings in the world, or maybe he does but only partially. I will try to illustrate this with *two examples* about how the child opens up to reality and to sadness.

Opening up to reality

The first example refers to the moment when T stands up in front of me, and it has to do with how he relates to external reality (his capacities). I observe how the child does not continue walking and does not grab my hands to be accompanied in his walks with the promptness and the ability that his motor skills might allow, because he cannot perceive himself and move in space. In the end, he freezes in a rigid and heavy posture. It is as if inside him there is no mental landscape, no cognitive map that he can project into his real experience in order to re-create it and make it become his own. I feel that I should not push him to walk, because "walking", as a symbolic activity, still does not belong to his internal world. At this point I feel that for T walking is still a premature activity, not because he is not physically unable to do it, but because he does not understand its sense, and I think that before doing it he should learn how to "experience space", to perceive himself as a subject in space.

Opening up to psychic pain

My second example has to do with sadness, which will become evident in the room every time the child looks at me or comes closer to me towards the end of the session; this emotion is characterised by a rich production of mucus and tears.

Unlike in the past, when we witnessed a dramatic reaction to my eyes, a persecutory, sudden reaction, like being stabbed in the middle of the forehead, followed by an incomprehensible whining, now the child cries in anguish, and his obstruction melts like a glacier: his tears flow copiously, as if a dam had burst. After the initial pain, of course, T reacts with irritation to this mucus, and would like to get rid of it, because he cannot stand it. If I try to help him wipe his nose, or dry his eyes, I immediately become a persecutor. Often, when we meet at the beginning of a session, as soon as he becomes aware of my presence he starts crying, as if he felt that I am the "cause" of a painful experience that he cannot tolerate, and he wants to send me away with his anguished crying. At the same time I observe that after giving vent to his pain with tears and mucus, T appears quite calm, relaxed and more alert; the parents had told me that his epileptic fits were often followed by such a reaction. We will have the opportunity to observe the sudden phenomenon of a clogged nose and of the sudden flow of mucus also in other patients. In the case of T, such a phenomenon dramatically appears for the first time on returning to therapy after a sudden interruption due to a mid-week festivity, and then starts reappearing almost automatically at the beginning or end of our sessions. This phenomenon will definitively disappear in the following months. Gradually, the child will be able to convey his sadness to me, and at the same time, to show me his joy, raising his arms and saying *"vava"*, allowing me to understand that he would like to drink some water.

In this period, the most significant aspect of T, from a developmental point of view, is the variation in the quality of his crying; for the first time I can hear an emotionally charged crying that conveys anguish, has the power of a calling and communicates an emotion. Similarly, when the child is calm, he is really present and serene, no longer detached and absent: he is with me. Together with the noises, also music will begin to find some space: a famous song by Ornella Vanoni, that says *"Tristezza per favore va' via tanto tu in casa mia no, non entrerai mai …"* ["Sadness, please go away, you will never get into my house anyway …"], which will become a refrain that I will often sing, attempting to alleviate his depression.

The call to life: beyond the VCR daddy

Thomas (seven years and four months)

He arrives in his mother's arms. He is sweet and smiling towards her. He lets me hold him in my arms without resisting. His back is straight but he seems to want to ignore me and does not return my greeting. However, he is perfectly aware of what is happening. As I briefly talk to his mother about the end of the therapy, she suddenly starts crying at the thought of what might happen the following autumn when his child will start going to primary school. As I try to comfort and reassure her, T starts grabbing my hair and opening his mouth as if he wanted to eat me without looking at me or being interested in my glasses. Then he starts rubbing one foot with the other, crossing his legs. I immediately tell him that he doesn't come to Doctor B to do physiotherapy.

In the therapy room, he sits comfortably on the couch, his hands on his sides as if they were armrests, and from that position starts banging his feet on the floor (he is big now and he can touch the floor) with an air of defiance. I wonder out loud as I approach him and sit beside him whether T is punishing me because he saw me talk to his mother and because he thinks that I am a bad doctor that makes his mother cry. He immediately stops banging on the floor and lies on my lap as usual. From his nesting position he kicks against the wall making a loud noise: the louder his blows, the more excited he seems. I look him in the eye with a stern expression letting him understand that I don't approve of his loud excitement and he stops for a few seconds. But then he changes his repertoire: he starts rubbing one foot with the other moving his bottom from one side to the other as if to dig a hole in the soft mattress. This activity is less noisy but much more irritating because it has a specific sexual, masturbatory meaning. He stops for a second just to see what my reaction would be, looking at me with a provocative expression. I tell him that he wants to challenge me today. He changes his repertoire again and starts playing with his hands and mouth, doing what—at this stage in the therapy—I call "the magic". I ask him to stop that accompanying my order with a light tap on his hand, saying: "ugly little hand". He stops suddenly and after a second he starts crying resentfully. I explain to him why I think he should not let himself be carried away by his magic. For five minutes he doesn't look at me and keeps his hands still along his sides. He seems to listen as I talk to him about my saying "no", which has become frequent in the last few weeks, towards his noisy or repetitive activities, as something that he rejects as bad. He looks quite resentful. Then, he starts looking at the lamp hanging from the ceiling, banging his feet and doing his "magic" with his mouth, accompanied by prolonged "te-te-te" sounds. I tell him that now he really wants to leave me and betray me with his lamp. He doesn't listen to me, so after a few minutes I feel that this excitement is taking him away not only from me but also from his body and himself, so I gently tap his cheek to make him understand that I am there and that I am interested in him, even if he pretends not to listen to me and even if he knows that I definitely disagree with what he is doing. At once, he stops his activity and resentfully tries to start crying again but with little success. After a while he comes down and re-establishes a contact even if his eyes are rather hostile and I feel that he is ready to start the challenge once again. Shortly after this, he starts rattling his teeth again and making a loud noise by banging his foot, which he holds in one hand, on the couch. I am surprised to see how powerfully stubborn he is in his ways.

Some fragile child! I ask him firmly, several times, to stop with his "magic". He stops for a while, but then he starts again. The seesaw of provocative behaviours goes on until the end of the session.

Thomas (seven years and six months)

He arrives held in his mother's arms (even if by now he is able to climb the stairs by himself, maybe with a little support). He whimpers, maybe because he has just been woken up, in the car. He has a bruise on his knee, but that is not the reason why he is whining. He lies on the mattress on the floor, but finds it difficult to keep his eyes open, as if he were very sleepy. He rattles his teeth and makes annoying sounds with his mouth. He stops only when I talk to him, commenting on his tiredness. For a few seconds he is agitated, kicks the chair and bangs his feet on the floor. He fills up the room with his noises, while from the outside comes the loud noise of the lorry collecting the rubbish from the dumpster bin. Then he unsuccessfully tries to sit up, so he stirs and stamps his feet.

With his right hand he grabs one of the soft cushions, brings it to his face and presses it against his mouth. He starts hitting it with his left hand, uttering a series of "te-te-te". He passes the cushion from one hand to the other. When he holds it in his left hand, he tends to put the right thumb into his mouth and suck its internal part. Instead, when he holds it in his right hand, he sucks the back of his left hand. He alternates these oral activities—or he accompanies them—with the banging of his feet against each other, or against the mattress. He cannot stop on anything, and he seems very excited. Then he lies down again, grabs the ends of the cushion with both hands and moves them closer, to make them meet in the middle, as he did, on other occasions, with his fists. He looks like a little boxer. He rubs the cushion on his lips, mumbles to it, then he loses it and looks for it in the air. He sits down again, placing the palm of his right hand on his mouth; then he turns it around, pushing its back against the lips with his left hand. I tell him that, today, with the "magic" of his hands and mouth he is forbidding me to get close to him. I add that what sets him against me is the fact that he knows that I am about to go away (it is almost summer, and therapy is going to stop soon), that I am going to close my room just as he is closing his mouth, and so he wants to tell me that he is no longer interested in my little songs, my hands and my eyes; he has decided to manage on his own, just as it happened with his mother, when she took her breast away from him when he was a baby. He stops and listens to me. He starts to stand up in order to go to his "nest", in his favourite position, which we know well: lying on my knees. With some effort he manages to reach the edge of the couch and he sits down. He starts banging his feet on the floor, going on like that until the end of the hour. His eyes are vigilant, and he makes me understand how he is aware of his complaint.

I move closer to him, ready to get his attention, as I did earlier with the soft tap on his cheek, in case I felt he is getting lost in his own noise. In the end I stand him up and I take him to the waiting room. Before being picked up by his mother, he still finds the time to powerfully grab my glasses. I notice that his aggressive gesture does not reduce the sense of estrangement and

alienation that in the last few months have accompanied our separations at the end of our sessions.

Commentary

What a struggle! What a struggle to acknowledge and respect the child, to keep appreciating the complexity of his experiences and to try to find some sense in his behaviours! What a struggle to reconcile in the mind my tender feelings towards him and his objective difficulties, and my angry feelings for his stubborn opposition to anything that might foster his development! What a struggle to tolerate the seesaw of feelings of despair (when, about two years from the beginning of therapy, no substantial changes in his relationships with objects and his own body can be seen) and of hope (when, in other moments, T seems able to be aware that he belongs to a world of shared meanings and to be with us without getting completely lost in the whirlwind of his self-excitement, his noisy motor stereotypies or being overwhelmed by the concreteness of his bodily experiences)! To this regard, I believe that nobody can miss the big difference between T's way of being inside the therapeutic experience and his body in the early sessions and in the conclusive period of the therapy. The child's attitude and behaviour have undergone important transformations: they appear to be the response of the child to a link with his therapist and the therapeutic context, which can be positive or oppositional, at times. The sensorial qualities, the forms of the scene and of the physical, bodily and human landscape in which he is immersed, have become—albeit in a partial and unstable manner—charged with emotional meaning. His being with me or against me is unequivocally different from the moments when he is far from me. A primitive distinction has been established between his Self and his body, and the Self and the body of his object, between his internal and external world, between the world of emotions and that of excitement, between communication and obsessional behaviour, between good dependence and tyrannical control.

In terms of reality, this means that T, now aged seven-and-a-half, is able to stand and to climb stairs with a little support; he can also make a few steps by himself, and seems to rely more willingly on people who are not his parents, like his physiotherapist and the teachers of his primary school. He has also kept an interest in spoken language, particularly in the music of language and music in general, which should comfort everyone. However, the burden of gloomy and heavy thoughts is inevitably still there, and it becomes intolerable if one thinks ahead and looks at his future and the developmental tasks awaiting him. In this sense one can understand his mother when she bursts into tears as she tries to imagine her child in a new school. It is significant that this pain can emerge just when she feels she can finally leave him in the hands of someone else and is able to see him a bit more autonomous and cooperative.

Final discussion

At the beginning of Chapter Five we wondered whether it was possible to interpret the behaviours of children and adolescents suffering from a pervasive developmental disorder, as we would interpret dreams, analysing the clinical material with the help of such notions as projective identification with part objects and the alpha function. Following Caccia's discussion (2012) on the distinction between primitive and psychotic, I made the hypothesis that the processes rooted in the early object relations with part objects, projective identification and the alpha function, showed particular characteristics in these patients, that the identification became intrusive and that the alpha function worked in reverse, thus causing an interruption or a pathological alteration or limitation of their mental development.

Such a hypothesis seems to find evidence in the clinical material, particularly when we observe Thomas as he turns into a "noisy war machine", or a "little Buddha", or when he stages his chaotic performances full of characters and sounds "on the stage of his mouth".

In such moments, anybody close to the child is overwhelmed by the paroxystic, sensual, and violent quality of his gestures, and by his absolute unwillingness to stop, to pause for a second and observe what he is doing with his body, hands, saliva, tongue and teeth, to listen to his body and to himself. Any observer discovers that the repeated and excited "performances" that he is forced to witness are not suitable to become metaphors of a link, as Bion might say; they are not suitable for communication (alpha elements) but only for evacuation, or the realisation of a delusional world (bizarre objects). Rarely can the observer have the impression to see through in transparency something known in T's "scripts", which he might have already noticed in very young children, thus believing that they might have a psychic meaning: a request for attention, ways to feel alive and powerful, a determination to listen or to accept orders.

In brief, whoever is near the child is faced with a "deaf and dumb physicality", apparently resistant to any concern or care, unavailable to any interaction or commonality (the "body" and the personifications that T represents through it appear to be either too evanescent and feeble, or too heavy and cumbersome). One wonders how it is possible to provide this body with a soul, to transform this "deaf and dumb" physicality into a piece of wood that can talk and feel: whether there might be, somewhere, a Mastro Geppetto or a "blue fairy" able to transform this Marionette-Thomas into a real child.

From this perspective, this clinical material is very interesting, because it confirms the hypothesis that the function of verbal language in children suffering from pervasive developmental disorder is absent or delayed, since the preverbal factors of language—dance, rhythm, laughing, and crying—are denied any possibility of being the expression of something that goes beyond the individual and that belongs instead to an identification with an Other, to something shared—as we saw in the interaction between "the little rascal and his mother", giving evidence of how this drama takes shape in a very precise place: the "theatre of the mouth".

We can therefore think that there is a close connection between the "deaf and dumb" body of T, the rambling performances of parts of his body inside and outside his mouth, and his serious difficulties with language. Although the child is able to understand what people tell him, or to guess its meaning, surely attracted by the tone and the rhythm of a sweet, melodious voice, he does not use verbal language to regulate closeness and distance from the Other, to ask for something, to cooperate in a task, to modify the surrounding world. He prefers to isolate himself in violent noises, in the din of his paroxystic movements or the harsh noises of saliva in his throat, rather than to communicate. Instead of crying, when frightened by a loud noise or an internal pain, he is struck dumb or starts whining.

CHAPTER SEVEN

Suzanne (S), a Goldilocks-like spiteful little girl: the growth of a new concept of self through the birth of imagination

Introduction

In this chapter, I will tell the story of Suzanne, a young girl who was about five and a half years old when she was referred to me for psychotherapy by the teacher of a special needs school in London specialised in the treatment of autistic children, which she had been attending for a few years. She suffered from spasticity and was severely delayed both verbally and non-verbally—according to the Reynell language test scale, her comprehension level was considered to be around the age of two years and seven months, whereas according to the Symbolic Play Test, her mental age was under twelve months. She showed several autistic features, such as lack of interest in interaction or communication with other people, immediate and delayed echolalia, and the tendency to become absorbed in simple and repetitive behaviours rather than playing with toys in a constructive way. In the special needs school, where she has recently passed from the last year of maternal school to the first year of primary school, she had always been considered as a difficult child, especially for the almost total lack of interest in what happened around her and what she was taught. S refused to talk to her teachers, to play with them or with the other children. Instead, she spent most of her time by herself and spoke a strange, completely incomprehensible jargon, a mixture of her native language—Spanish and English, but without any grammatical structure. Sometimes she asked to go to the toilet, where she would spend hours mumbling and looking inside the toilet bowl, fascinated by the flushing water.

In that period, towards the end of the 1970s and the beginning of the 1980s, I was in London for my training in Child Psychotherapy and I worked in a Child Guidance Clinic in the city centre. Here, I was able to see the child for psychoanalytic psychotherapy four times a week for about a year until her parents, both from South America, decided to go back to their country of origin. At the same time, having much free time as a training student, I was able to write the detailed notes of all the sessions. In doing this, I was stimulated by my participation in a workshop on psychotherapy for mentally handicapped patients, both children and adults, organised by Dr Neville Symington in the adult department of the Tavistock clinic. In this research space, I was encouraged by my colleagues to start psychotherapy with a child like S, apparently quite damaged both neurologically and cognitively. In those years, very little was known from a psychoanalytical viewpoint (Clarke, 1933; Mannoni, 1964 [1972]; Symington, 1981) about the development of personality of this kind of patients and the possibility of analysing them, even if Melanie Klein (1927, 1931, 1946), studying the inhibitions and the delays in the symbolic development of children, had stated that some forms of mental retardation had to be considered as disguised psychoses.

The choice of starting psychotherapy with S was also motivated by my previous experiences as a neurologist in rehabilitation and educational institutions, where I had seen many children who were suffering from spasticity, epilepsy, learning or physical disabilities, due to metabolic or genetic illnesses, who, apart from their specific problems, also showed very serious emotional and behavioural difficulties. In those contexts, I was aware of the great suffering in their internal world which remained silent and unheard, since the most primitive aspects of their behaviour, due to the lack of specific technical knowledge, were labelled tout court as "delay" and since nobody had the courage to seek an emotional contact with their life experience which was apparently very limited and to offer them a personal space in which an intimate relationship could develop.

You might wonder why I wanted to discuss the clinical case of S at this point in the book. The answer is simple. From a developmental point of view, this child seems to take over from Thomas, in the sense that the structure of her personality at the beginning of therapy was very similar to Thomas' personality structure at the end of his therapy. This will allow us to analyse the phenomenology of her infantile transference as the expression of a mental and emotional functioning slightly more evolved than Thomas'. We will see how, in her external and internal relationships, unlike what we have observed in Thomas, the flow of identifications with part and whole objects, which constitute the *physiology* of the early object relations (Caccia, 2012) was quite recognisable but at the same time desperately searching for a mind capable of containing and transforming it. If in the case of the previous patient the main function of the therapist's reverie was to give a shape and a name to his emotional and physical experiences, in the case of S its main function was to fit them into a context, in a mental landscape of shared meanings.

The organisation of this chapter has a traditional structure. In the first part, I will try to highlight the complexity of the child's experience, development and personality. In the second part, I will describe the therapeutic experience as it developed from the beginning to the end, choosing the most significant sequence from the material from a development point of view. In the third and last part, I will present my reflections on the material itself and on my countertransference experience.

Clinical history

S was the only child of a couple of Argentinian immigrants who had lived and worked in England for many years. She was born prematurely at thirty weeks and she weighed a little more than one-and-a-half kilo. While she was hospitalised in the intensive care unit, she suffered from several cyanotic fits and a pathological jaundice for which she had to undergo a complete blood transfusion. She was discharged in an apparently normal state, even if she was still in the list of children at risk and was a very calm baby at home. She was fed with artificial milk and she never showed any particular liveliness. For this reason she was treated by her parents as a fragile object, with great care and apprehension.

At the age of eight months, her mother noticed that she kept her hands fisted and after a neurological check the child was diagnosed with spastic quadriplegia, without epileptic complications. From then on, S started attending a centre for spastic children regularly, where she was offered session of physiotherapy and speech therapy and, until the age of two, she made great progress both in motor skills and verbal language. For a brief period, everyone thought that she would develop well and started hoping that she would soon walk by herself and catch up also in the area of verbal language. Unfortunately however, as soon as S started attending a children centre once a week, all these hopes vanished. The teachers immediately noticed that the child did not play in an industrious and expressive manner; on the contrary, she would always play with the same toy, banging it on the floor and making some noise. In the same period, S became less cooperative in psychological tests and started to mumble on her own, using a special language in which one could recognise a mixture of English and Spanish words. She also started to constantly repeat the same words like the name of her physiotherapy, "child" and "bye-bye".

At the age of three she started attending kindergarten. After an initial positive period during which she learned to be more autonomous, to eat and drink by herself, and to be potty trained, her development stopped. In the two years that followed, she made no progress; indeed, her ability to focus on things progressively decreased. She increasingly refused to look people in the eye, to the point that she even began to avoid looking at herself in the mirror. More often and for longer periods of time she kept talking only in her incomprehensible language, laughing to herself in an inappropriate manner, and withdrawing in herself, lying on a table or sinking into her armchair. It was assumed that she might suffer from a mild form of epileptic *petit mal*, but when repeated EEG scans proved negative, there were no more doubts that her difficulties in getting in touch with people and her scarce motivation were the signs of a deeper emotional disorder.

The parents

What immediately struck me about S's parents, whom I met several times during the consultation period, was the extreme precision of their memories of the child's life and the descriptions of her behaviours.

The mother, who was always the more active of the two in our meetings, kept comparing her experience of her daughter with that of a one-year-old child whom she looked after as a baby-sitter. She told me that she could not believe that such a young child could be so curious, interested, and gratifying, so ready to interact with her. He was completely different from her daughter, who was, instead, rejecting, uncooperative, capricious, never accepting anything that was offered to her, never affectionate, often distant, isolated, and withdrawn. The mother added that, in the light of her experience as a nanny, she was disappointed, confused, and unable to find an explanation for what was happening between the two of them; she became convinced that her daughter was *stupid and bad*.

The parents also told me that S still did not speak in the first person and that—especially before falling asleep—*she spent hours repeating, like a tape recorder, everything her mother had told her during the day*. When she was hungry, she would scream and cry desperately: she could not bear to wait, or to receive something that was different from what she was expecting. Sometimes she would also throw away something that she had tenaciously asked for, saying, "*You do not want it*". Then she would start crying desperately, as if someone had purposely taken it away from her.

She sometimes cried for a long time even during the day, apparently with no reason. Other times, before going to bed in the evening, she would hit her favourite doll, saying, "*Cry, cry*". Then she would start crying herself, going on for quite a while, without any possibility of being comforted. On those occasions, she refused to listen to her mother and even chased her away. Thus, she would often end up in tears, in her little room, completely alone and abandoned.

On the whole, the child's clinical history and the parents' narrative made me think about how difficult it was for S to interact with other children (every time she joined a group of children, she had withdrawn in herself after an initial moment of openness), and to manage to remain in her real skin as a child without resorting—in difficult moments like going to sleep or waiting for food—to a false identity, supported by processes of projective and adhesive identification with damaged internal objects that are punitive ("you don't want it"), detached ("the tape recorder"), and confused with the omnipotent aspects of her infantile Self.

The therapeutic experience

Diagnostic sessions

The proper beginning of therapy was preceded by a series of preliminary assessment meetings, during which I was able to ascertain how difficult it was for the child to separate from her mother and remain alone in the company of a person—and a context—that she did not know.

S had a rather robust build, even if at a superficial glance she might look smaller than her peers, since spasticity prevented her from standing straight. Either standing or sitting, she tended to crumple up and lean forwards. She would move her head around in all directions, while her body remained rigid and unstable. She had a sweet face, deep, dark eyes which sometimes lit up with curiosity and happiness, and dark, smooth, and thick hair which made her look rather pretty and attractive. Her parents, too, were two beautiful young people.

In her relationship with me and the clinic environment, S immediately showed a puzzling behaviour. Every time I went to the waiting room to meet her, she welcomed me with a big smile and started moving about with her whole body, as if she could not wait to end up in my arms. As we descended the two ramps of stairs leading to the therapy room on the ground floor, she rested her head on my shoulder and in silence she carefully watched everything around her. To reassure her, I talked to her about the spaces we were going through, anticipating the obstacles (doors, steps) that we would encounter, and I showed her the lights on the ceiling that shone on our path, just as I would do with a much younger child. All this made her feel contained.

However, as soon as we entered the therapy room, this fragile equilibrium was shattered: the moment I sat her in the small soft armchair which I had placed for her near the doll house, S's reaction was catastrophic, as if she felt completely lost and abandoned. At first she burst into tears, inconsolably crying, and then she slid off the armchair and lay on the floor in a foetal position; or she sat and stared at the light from the window, crying all the time. *There was no way of comforting her.* She was unreachable in her desperation. Only by gently calling S by her name could I sometimes make her stop crying and remain silent for a very little while; otherwise, it was a real tragedy. Because of this, on more than one occasion, I had to ask her mother to join us in the therapy room and stay with us during our sessions. The mere presence of S's mother seemed to immediately calm her down; but it also had the effect of definitively distancing her from me, as one can see in the material of the last assessment session, after which I decided to start intensive psychotherapy with her.

As soon as I closed the therapy room S began to cry and scream desperately as I placed her in the soft armchair near the doll's house, on the right of the entrance door. I sat next to S to reassure her, and I tried to talk to her, telling her that there was nothing for her to fear. I tried to attract her attention by calling her by her name, uselessly. She seemed unable to hear me. After ten minutes of this tragedy I asked her mother to join us in the room. Following my invitation, the mother sat on my chair (which from now on I will call "the big chair") beside my desk, on which a lamp was lit. At the sight of her mother S calmed down immediately and allowed me to help her stand up in order to get closer to the doll's house. She started to touch several items in it: first the toy bathtub and the toilet, then the little girl-doll. After this she started undressing her, as if she wanted to give her a bath. She said "filth" several times. She named the toys and other items in the doll's house, but without inviting me to take part in her game. A few times she interrupted her mumbling and her touching the objects only to look towards an indefinite point above my head, in the direction of her mother, who was sitting silently behind me. Then she grabbed the toy wardrobe from the doll's house. After sitting on the carpet next to me S tried hard to open it, as if she were looking for something to eat. At this point her mother left the room without saying anything. As soon as the child realised that the "big chair" was "empty", she dropped the toy wardrobe and burst into tears. Then she stared at the brightly lit window. Her eyes, still wet with tears, were dim and lifeless, and the balance of her body was unstable. After a while she lay on the floor in a foetal position: motionless, with a finger in her mouth, she seemed to be wrapped inside a cocoon. I called her by her name several times, to "wake her up from her torpor", until she turned her eyes towards me. She then picked up the toy wardrobe and rubbed it on the floor and on my foot, after which she burst into tears once again. A little later she stopped crying. I did not understand why she had calmed down, whether because she was tired or resigned, but I heard some rumbling noises coming from her body, and I saw that she was grimacing in pain. At the same time I noticed that she was finding it hard to swallow her saliva. A few seconds later, now completely awake, she made me understand that she wanted to stand up, so I gave her a hand. At first she moved towards the "big empty chair" near the desk, where her mother had sat, and then she went back towards the door, where she stopped for a few minutes, motionless, resting her back against my hand. Then she threw her head backwards and looked at the empty chair and at the lamp on the desk once again. When she moved her head back in its proper position, she stared at me intensely, letting me know that she wanted to get out of the room. This was the first time that I became a somewhat interesting object for her […].

Commentary

In this session it is possible to notice how in the absence of the real mother S is invaded by an unspeakable anxiety. She tries with all her might to oppose this new situation, crying and screaming almost to the point of collapsing. Alternatively, she isolates herself completely: she fixedly stares at the light from the window, or she slides onto the floor, where she lies in a foetal position.

Unlike T (with his whining), with her cries, screams, and regressive behaviour, seems to be able to convey her anxieties, fear and anger to those near her. She also seems very tenacious when she tries to impose her will and fulfil her wishes, albeit limited and restricted, and to open her eyes to reality when she is called by her name.

Another surprising factor is her slow walk around the room at the end of the session, first in the direction of the "big chair" and the lamp, and then towards the door. The child repeats exactly what her mother did half an hour earlier. *I wonder in which mysterious way S was able to register the details of the earlier scene in which her mother had been the protagonist, lost as she was in her drama.* This skill of hers reminds one of what happens to her in bed in the evening, when she repeats like a tape recorder everything that her mother said to her during the day.

Also in her use of the various toys, particularly the tub and the wardrobe of the doll house, S reveals something peculiar: she treats them as if they were real, life-size ones, like those that she uses at home. She seems to think that she could really have a bath in the toy tub, or that she could find a drawer full of food inside the wardrobe, and she gets very angry when these wishes do not come true.

To me, she is like a little *Alice in Wonderland* that does not how to get out of the bad room in which she has fallen. *Just like Alice, she cannot find the right size for herself or her things*: either she is too small for the objects that surround her (having drunk from the bottle whose label says "drink me") or because she is too big (having eaten the pastry whose label says "eat me")! In her experience of identity the "as if" dimension is replaced by a concrete thought, and the distinction between internal and external is unstable and tends to disappear.

However, among all her behaviours during this session, the most striking one is her sudden "awakening": within a few seconds, S re-establishes a contact with me on a reality level; she leaves the persecutory state in which she had fallen and asks me to help her stand up and support her with my hand as she starts her little walk towards the door of the therapy room. After being for her the White Rabbit of Alice's dream, who took her to the bad therapy room, I suddenly become the "doctor who can open and close doors", who can "take her to, or away from, her mother". What magic has modified her state of conscience?

Have we really ended up in the world of the Reverend mathematician Charles Dodgson, aka Lewis Carroll?

The beginnings of therapy

Proper therapy started a few months later, after a long pause, and the sessions were soon organised according to an unchanging script:

1. In the waiting room the child usually greeted me with joy and excitement. She moved about, as if she were impatient to come into my arms, and she readily reacted to my gaze.
2. Once in my arms, as I walked along the corridor towards the stairs, she immediately grabbed my hair, pulling it down with some strength. Then she moved her open mouth closer to my head or my cheek, as if wanting to eat me (this "as if" activity was very realistic, even if it had a transference meaning). However, there was no need for me to defend myself from such voracious and aggressive gestures, because immediately after that she always established a physical contact with my hair and my face, which was warm, tender, and loving.
3. Once in the therapy room she no longer cried; instead, she immediately looked at the "big chair", where her mother had sat in the past. If I talked to S about her fear and sadness, of being alone without her mummy, she pretended nothing was happening.
4. Once on the floor, she immediately headed for the doll house; there, she first touched the toys, and then she played with the doll, the water sink and the bath tub. She undressed the doll, washed or fed her, quickly passing from one action to the next in a mechanical and repetitive way, accompanying her gestures with some verbal comments in her favourite jargon. Her play activity merely seemed to be the repetition or re-visitation of fragments of her real experience, but with a particular characteristic: at times she seemed unable to differentiate the doll from herself, reality from fantasy.
5. Often, as a consequence of the intrusive noises from the street outside, or from inside her own body, she stopped playing and dropped

on the floor, where she crumpled up and took the toys to her mouth as if they were food, isolating herself from everything.

6. She alternated this activity with moments in which she turned her eyes to the brightly lit window at the other end of the room, opposite the entrance. Staring at the window, she smiled or laughed excitedly on her own, repeating to herself the words "I love you more" endlessly, without any contact with me. In this state of isolation, she seemed to be absorbed in a completely private experience, in which she seemed *to enjoy a special and blissful relationship with an imaginary object, or to be lost into an idealised womb-object.*
7. These moments of elation did not last long: soon S burst into desperate crying, or she started to take everything to her mouth, while the pain in her stomach increased. In the end she looked hungry and exhausted. Crumpled up on the floor, with the little energy that was left, she silently tried hard to get her hands into the wardrobe of the doll's house in search for food.
8. As for her verbal activity, S named most of the objects that she touched or got hold of with a flat and mechanical tone of voice, always using a mixture of English and Spanish words.

Commentary

From these notes we can first of all see the great instability of the child's internal world: her attitude towards the object changes suddenly. Her mood swings (from excited to depressed and vice versa) are continuous and intense, just like the direction of her attention (from external to internal, and vice versa). At the same time we notice that also the distinction between reality and fantasy is not so certain: the "as if" quality of her play is often annihilated by the wish or the urgency of a need. This might be interpreted as the consequence of a very primitive infantile transference with the toy, to the point that S for example, is no longer able to see the difference between the doll and herself, really believing that in the drawer from the doll's house she can find the real food that she is desperately looking for.

Finally the similarity between the quality of her play and her way of naming the toys is striking: both activities, in their repetitiveness, seem to hinder communication; they seem to have the same function of T.'s "war machine" behaviours: to give a certain tone and sense of importance to the child, being the expression of a desperate solipsistic performance, which cannot tolerate any pauses or breaks. She repeats and does not invent, and in repeating she feels she exists. Her imitations are merely instrumental, not pleasant. In addition to this, we can observe that *in her play or speech there are no contexts or landscapes that can be used to construct a story.*

In her relationship with people and their bodies, S seems, instead, to have access to a more three-dimensional world; for example, when she utters somebody's first name, often repeating it a thousand times, she does it in a sweet, melodious manner. Apparently, the first names of the people she is fond of seem to arouse pleasant associations and memories in her mind, resonating and finding a space in her internal world (and maybe that is why I have chosen to help her, from the very beginning, to get out her states of isolation by calling her by her name). It is easy to compare S's behaviours to those of T—although they were much more evanescent and feeble—and at the same time to wonder about the meaning of their behaviours: are they really the expression—albeit primitive—of an aesthetic experience similar to that of a baby who is taken in and captured by the beauty of her object, or are they the manifestation of an envious act of stealing or of an adhesive identification with the object, so that the two children, after furtively getting hold of the name, can wrap themselves into the melodious sound of its syllables?

In Chapter Ten we will see Al play in a similar manner with the accent of his Roman dialect and with the word "indaco" (indigo).

The first period of therapy: the spiteful child

About halfway through the first three months of therapy, S missed a session because she was ill. The following week she came to me accompanied only by her father. The combination of two factors—the missed session and the absence of her mother—were probably very significant in terms of the material that followed.

> As soon as I picked her up S started to pull my hair so violently that her father, who was witnessing the scene, became quite anxious. Then she started opening her mouth, as if wanting to eat my head and face. Immediately after that, when we were still in the corridor, she called out "mummy" for the first time and she rested her little face on my cheek. In the room, after a few timid attempts at playing with the toys, washing the little doll

and her hair, S dropped on the floor, lay on one side, in a foetal position and angrily started biting the little doll and her clothes. She seemed disappointed because she had not been "really" able to wash the doll's hair. She did not utter a single word in English, and she kept mumbling incomprehensible words in Spanish. I talked to her about the missed session and the absence of her mother; in response to this, she suddenly sat up and started singing "If you're happy and you know it, clap your hands". A few minutes later, with some effort, she crawled towards the large wardrobe next to the "big chair" and unsuccessfully tried to open it several times. She then saw a bag full of wooden blocks in a corner of the room, which I had prepared to make her play. She put her hands into the bag, as if she was looking for something to eat. As soon as she realised that the bag only contained wooden blocks she got angry, threw everything away and lay down, with her belly on the floor. Then she rolled away from me, towards the middle of the room, where she remained motionless, all curled up, alternating moments of silence with shrill shrieks. I asked her what was happening, but she did not answer. I moved closer to her, trying to capture her eyes, but she absolutely avoided eye contact with me, clearly showing me that she wanted to be left alone. I noticed that she was playing with the saliva in her mouth, so I talked to her about her anger towards me, because I did not allow her to open the wardrobe and touch or take the other children's toys. I added that perhaps she was thinking that I was hiding something very precious in the wardrobe, my best food for the other children, while I had only taken out a bag of wooden blocks for her. I tried to make her understand how jealous she was of the other children, and how she felt rejected by me. At this point she started to speak in English and to tell me—frequently repeating the same sentences and words—the story of a family of bears (daddy bear, mummy bear, and baby bear) and of a very hungry and spiteful young girl who got lost in the woods and was able, at dinnertime, to furtively get into their house and eat the sweet of the baby bear, without being seen.

Commentary

For the first time the child expresses herself appropriately, using only the English language. She wants to tell me a fairy tale.

I feel that something has pushed her out of the usual script, "if you're happy and you know it, clap your hands!" She seemed to have understood my interpretation, when I talked to her about her envy of the other children's food, without a manic reaction on her part. To my great surprise, she shows no urgency to simply take centre-stage and she tells me a story whose content and characters have triggered important identifications in her: a story that talks about other characters, which has, somehow, partly become her own story. At once I perceive her fairy story as a dream that contains something very deep and personal about her, which is linked to her infantile experiences of being a lonely and "hungry" child.

Beyond the contents, an important aspect of this interaction is that the development and unfolding of the narrative is the result of a shared effort: on one hand, she absolutely wants me to pull me into her story, and on the other I, not knowing the tale, must ask her several times to stop, to repeat what she is telling me and to be more precise in her links, especially where the context and the landscape of the characters become confused. My attitude towards her words and images becomes progressively more similar to the one I have towards the dreams of my patients, when we try together to "complete the scene" of the internal drama which has found its first expression in the dream images that they have offered me. Against any expectation on my part, she accepts to help me understand her and to be helped to express herself. My attempts to interpret what she is telling me are progressively supported by a dream of mine, which has to do with her behaviour in the therapy room and of which she is the main character, just as the spiteful girl is the protagonist of the fairy tale.

After the session, talking to my English colleagues in the clinic, I have discovered that S's story has to do with one of the most famous fairy tales for children in England: "The story of Goldilocks and the three bears". In a later meeting with her parents, I have also learned that for several weeks now S has kept asking her mother to read her this particular story before going to bed, and that she enjoys laughing maliciously particularly when Goldilocks furtively eats the sweet of the little bear.

In the following session:

> I immediately noticed that the child was very vigilant. As soon as she entered the room she looked at the two lamps hanging from the ceiling above our heads. She stared at them for a long time, mumbling to herself, while I was thinking about the light in the bears' house (in the fairy tale) she had told me in our previous session. She played with the doll's house as usual, and she dropped the little doll. Then she took the bag with the wooden blocks and threw it away with contempt. Finally she focused on the

big wardrobe, clearly intending to open it. Silently, she dropped on the floor next to the wardrobe and with a sly expression tried to force it open from below. She looked me in the eye several times, with a provoking smile. She gave me the impression that she knew very well that she was being spiteful towards me. I talked to her about her curiosity to know what was inside the wardrobe and of her wish to take the food and the toys of the other children, just as Goldilocks did with the food of the little bear. At this point, just as the shrill cry of a young child from the street under our window was heard, she felt a sharp and sudden pain in her stomach. I tried to understand whether she had heard the voice of the child, but she did not pay attention to what I was asking her and asked to be helped to stand up. She moved closer to me and after briefly looking at the window in silence, she started playing with my glasses. She pulled them down to the tip of my nose looking at me and then started laughing. After that, she got hold of them and played with them for a while, opening and closing them. She unsuccessfully tried to put them on, and finally started biting and sucking them. With some effort, I managed to take them back.

At this point, no longer interested in my glasses, she moved even closer to my body and started exploring my chest. She looked into my jumper, making sucking noises with her mouth, as if she were looking for breasts. Then she lay face down on my leg. While she was lying there, all crumpled up, she felt a sharp pain in her stomach. Thinking that it might be due to her position, I tried to help her lie down more comfortably, but she thanked me with a bite. In the end, after playing with my glasses a bit more, she let herself fall down, this time away from me, looking very disappointed. She picked up the little doll that she had dropped on the floor at the beginning of the session and started sucking it and biting its clothes as if they were food. Then she did the same to her hands. At this point I told her that she was a little Goldilocks, and that she was angry with me; for her, I had become a bad-daddy-bear that prevented her from getting the food or the toys of the other children-bears from the wardrobe. I made her notice that our room was lit, just like the house of the bear family. I also told her that, by stealing my glasses, she might want to take my place as the "master of the house", just as she sometimes might want to get hold of the breasts and the body of her mother, whom she felt full of dangerous babies, like those who were passing and shouting under our window. I added that she was very jealous of the fact that in this period her mother was looking after another baby, and she was afraid that he might take mummy's breast and milk away from her, leaving her hungry, or that he might occupy mummy's belly, a place where she always wanted to go back to. For the second time I had the impression that S was interested in my words: she stopped "eating" the doll and once again, attentively, looked at the two lamps hanging from the ceiling. Without telling her anything, I thought that the two lit lamps were like two eyes that shone on her internal world, and that our brightly lit room was like the kitchen of the bear house in the tale, a place where she could get in and stay without too much fear [...].

Commentary

The material of these sessions shows the importance of the episode in which the child, through the fairy tale, unconsciously suggested a story that allowed me to gather her behaviours, movements and actions into a single unifying image, and to start exploring their emotional meaning.

I cannot say to what extent my attempt to convey to her a picture of her experience within the therapeutic context through the metaphor of the fairy tale may have helped S to increase her Self-awareness. Certainly, however, it has allowed her to feel contained, thought about, understood, and above all relieved, realising that in front of her there was a mind that no longer saw her behaviours as "negative" events resulting from her stupidity and badness. At the same time, I believe that S felt quite relieved seeing that I acknowledged not only her anxieties and fears towards me and the room, but also her greedy and overbearing infantile parts without being frightened by them. Moreover, it was very important for me to discover, with some surprise, that S her own internal resources which could help her get in touch with her deepest emotional experiences—or, at least, that a certain impulse was still alive in her, i.e., to search in her external reality, just as in the tale of Goldilocks, for something that could give shape to her internal world. This awareness led me to avoid physical contact with her to reduce her tendency to go back to concrete modalities of exchange. For example, I began to help her go down the stairs holding her hand and no longer holding her in my arms. At the same time I tried to find a way to favour the flow of her more primitive identifications, reducing my interpretations of the likely meaning of her behaviour, providing her, instead, with images of how she represented herself within the therapeutic experience.

After the episode of the fairy tale of Goldilocks and the technical modifications I have described, the "script" of the sessions changed. The child abandoned for good the area of the room with the soft armchair, the big wardrobe and the doll's house. She decided, instead, to sit on the large chair next to the writing desk with the lamp, the telephone and the Yellow Pages directory, and she started to play the "game of the great big lady".

The second period of therapy: the great big lady

The fact that the change of script took place on the occasion of the first interruption of therapy, during the Christmas holidays, is quite significant.

S started a new activity, or rather, she changed the subject of her performance, choosing another character and a different stage: she moved towards the "big chair", demanded to use it and sit on it, to have the Yellow Pages directory available and to play with the telephone on my desk. I told her that the chair on which she now sat belonged to "the grownups", i.e., her mother and myself, and that she wanted to be a "big lady", like us. She smiled at me. She spent most of the following sessions sitting on the "big chair", turning the Yellow Pages, naming the objects that she recognised there, and trying to make a few phone calls. The quality of these activities was not so different from her playing with toys, if not for the fact that *the confusion here was mainly about her identity*, and not about the contents of what she was doing. In the past, the pretend act of giving a bath to the little doll lost its quality of a play activity and was confused with the real act of giving a bath to a child (a symbolic equation). Now, it was the personification with the "great big lady" that was no longer easily distinguishable from "being the big lady". Her processes of identification with the object led to an absolute (or almost absolute) disappearance of the child's own Self, and above *all of her infantile true Self.*

The main consequence of this state of things was that, if her activities on the chair and at the desk were interrupted by the noises coming from outside the clinic, by some physical pain inside the child's body or by the oncoming evening darkness, S was overwhelmed by anxiety or uncontainable anger, and she started to take anything to her mouth: the pages of the book, or the phone receiver. She was once again a small, paralysed and terrified child; for the same reasons, in the past, she stopped playing with her toys and started biting and chewing the little doll and its clothes. The intensity and concreteness of these regressive moments became increasingly stronger as we approached the first break in the analysis, and on some occasions they became manifest as the child's negative reaction to my voice, my words and my English, especially when I tried to talk to her about our imminent separation. I noticed, however, something quite new, compared to the past: eventually, after calling her by her name, to make her direct her gaze towards me, she was able to look at me, as if she were now capable of keeping a separation between the "good" upper part of my face (the eyes, the glasses and the hair that she could grasp or attack without feeling too persecuted), and the lower part, which she experienced as bad (the mouth, the sound and the saliva which terrified her).

Of course, back from the Christmas holidays, S showed even more determination to play the part of the "great big lady" or sitting on my chair, with the telephone and the Yellow Pages. She rejected all the other toys, or more suitable books, throwing them on the floor, just as she had done earlier with the bag full of building blocks. At the same time, she started to attack me more directly, farting and chanting on top of my voice, mostly speaking in Spanish and transforming her speech in a "salad of words". She clearly conveyed to me that I should not dare to challenge her conviction of really being "the great big lady" of the situation: reading from the book, sitting in the "big chair", dialling telephone numbers, and even farting, meant being in control of her object, of me and of the whole world, pretending to know everything and to need nothing. I was irritated and unhappy, and on several occasions I thought I could lose my temper or give up the struggle to make her come down to earth, especially in those moments when S *showed greater interest in listening to the rustling sound of the Yellow Pages than to my words*.

These feelings were further exasperated by a general difficulty in understanding what processes might support her sense of identity and her behaviour: was it projective identification, adhesive identification or some undetected brain damage? At first I thought that this repeated, painful experience of being ignored by the "the great big lady", which made me feel helplessly sorry and angry, was something that belonged to her: maybe she, too, at her infantile level, experienced the same feelings towards our adult world. But then, thinking about the quality of her actions, I started to see that her "being over the top" was accomplished through a very primitive, two-dimensional way of reading the Yellow Pages, and that her attempts at understanding, through the book's images, what the world was like and how relationships worked between people and things, led her to erroneous or limited conclusions.

To this regard, I talked to her a great deal about her view of mummy and daddy, or the therapist, when they were on the phone or reading the Yellow Pages, whom she tried hard to imitate, to make her notice how through her imitation she became a very "busy" child, who should not be disturbed, just as she experienced her parents and me as very "busy".

Thus, I began to show more interest in her "readings", and I talked to her about her attempts to put some order in the chaos she found herself in, when she looked at the images and the letter of the words in the Yellow Pages, and of her wish to understand and get access to the difficult and mysterious reality of the private life of her parents and therapist, and of their bodies. Thus, the letters became babies, penises, food and poo, noises and words with different qualities, while the book became the mind, belly, breast, bottom and genitals of her objects and of herself.

In brief, I tried to survive, somehow, her attempt at annihilating my presence in her life inside the therapy room, and to find some opening in her general "no entry" attitude, which, in any case, was qualitatively different from the moments of catastrophic isolation of the earlier periods of therapy.

Spaces and intervals

All these efforts gradually led to important shifts in the child's development. There were big changes in her motor behaviour in the course of the sessions. S became more capable of controlling her body and her posture: she stopped slumping like a bag of potatoes and learned to sit on the "big chair". In particular, she started to move around with greater freedom, exploring the room, reaching for new objects and moving closer, or away from me. I noticed that her better mastery over her body allowed S to discover "the spaces" between it and the other objects. The first space that she discovered was the one between her body and the desk when she sat on the "big chair". Then she discovered her own image reflected in my glasses, realising that what she saw there was her own face.

At the same time she also became more aware of the "intervals" between sessions, times, and place, which meant being separated from me and from other people. When she felt very anxious about external noises or frightened by my voice she was even able to ask me: "Is time up?"-"Going home now?" It was as if my voice had become "bad", since it was associated with the end of the session and with being "sent away".

Separation became a more understandable and containable experience for S even if she still tended to express her feelings at a very primitive level. For example, when her favourite teacher was away for a whole week halfway during the term, S refused to go to school, cried every morning before leaving home and wetted her bed at night. Moreover, her mother told me that the child had started drawing my face when she was at home. She also wanted to draw the faces of other people she knew, and she was able to distinguish them.

Moving towards the children's area

Together with these new achievements, S spontaneously left the area of the "big chair" and started playing under the window, in the brighter part of the room, where there had always been a small chair and a small table for children, which she had always ignored. The movement towards the children's area was characterised by the appearance of a new "script".

Sitting straight on her little chair, with her hands on the small table, S began to spend quite some time in activities that mainly involved her mouth and hands: she did not play with toys, but with her own body, alternating oral activities, like sucking her tongue or grinding her teeth, with other actions like hitting and stroking the table or my hands, to strike them or use them as a soft cushion on which to rest. I thought that S was busy trying through very primitive experiments to understand the difference between soft and hard, empty and full, inside and outside her body, as a normal baby would do. For the first time she made me feel very sorry for her, because she seemed to be terribly small and vulnerable, and she was not alienated in her relationship with me.

The last period of therapy: a premature conclusion

The last period of therapy was sad and depressing. The Easter holidays had a deep emotional impact on the child. When we met again after the break.

S, initially, showed her great joy in seeing me again, but once in the room her mood changed, and she became glum and confused. She was unable to recognise the things around her or to get in touch with me, as if during the break she had lost the ability to remember and to select those objects in the room which had become important for both of us in the course of our therapeutic experience.

She noticed the two lamps on the ceiling and the "big chair" only after quite some time. I talked to her about what those objects might have represented for us, and this helped her to find them inside herself. Then, gradually and with much help, she remembered the other things as well. The end of the session was rather dramatic. She threw on the floor all the toys that we had just brought back to memory, showing how powerful her anger was in damaging her ability to remember and to introject her experiences. She spared only the little doll, of which she was very fond, and that on many occasions had stood for herself. Before going out, she left it on the edge of the table, in a very precarious position.

After a few sessions, the parents told me that the following autumn they would go back to their native country. Thus, I started working with S with the intention of stopping just before the summer. Our sessions became difficult and repetitive, and started following the old "scripts". At first the child would cry desperately, calling for her mummy or daddy; then, after calming down, she would play the part of one of her favourite characters—often "the great big lady"—cutting me off completely and using language only to order and command.

I became aware the S tended to repeat with me the same behaviour that she had with her mother at home; thus, I decided to pay more attention to the level of her development, allowing her to express her feelings without forcing her attention with my interpretations. I felt that despite her anger and despair she was not isolated in a world of her own; instead, she was present in the session, and she used me as a container for her most unpleasant experiences.

With just a few moments of softer, tender, affectionate contact, the therapy reached its conclusion very quickly. In the end, I was left with the feeling of great uselessness in terms of the work that had been done; however, when I saw S again after the summer for a review session, I had a different impression: the child seemed to be less rejecting, sang me two songs that she had learned at school, and when she went back to her parents at the end of the session, S kept following me with her eyes until she disappeared at the end of the corridor.

The therapeutic functions

At this point I will try to describe some of the therapeutic functions of containment and interpretation that I think I have carried out in my relationship with S. In this way, I hope that the nature of the child's experience in the therapy room will become clearer: what changes may have taken place in her and what may have determined them. For this purpose, I would like to illustrate three important developmental steps, each of which coincided with a different way used by the child to explore the play room and my body.

In the course of therapy, the play room was divided by S in three different areas:

A. The area of the soft armchair, the big wardrobe and the doll's house.
B. The area of the big chair and the desk with a lamp, the telephone and the Yellow Pages book.
C. The children's area, with small chairs and a small table, in the brighter part of the room.

In these spaces, in different moments of the therapeutic process, S expressed different ways of relating to me and to herself.

In the first space, the child did not seem able to maintain a significant contact with reality, nor to establish an emotional link with me, or part of me. Her play activity and her language were repetitive, and they mainly worked as a defence from deep persecutory anxieties. The moments when she was able to get out of her states of isolation and faced reality, were characterised by a spasmodic search for something to put in her mouth, to chase away every discomfort or pain, just like milk for a baby.

In the second space S alternated moments in which she put herself in the "great big lady's shoes" and others when she became a little, frightened baby who sucked everything around her. The purpose of her being "the great big lady", as I have said before, was to convey, albeit in a primitive way, her internal relationship with a primary maternal object.

Finally, in the third space, the so-called "children's area", S looked very vulnerable; she alternated her explorations of the table-hand-breast with activities of auto-erotic, mainly oral, nature. The child seemed to be looking for very primitive physical sensations, like hardness and softness, attempting to differentiate internal and external spaces, as if she were a new-born-baby, or only a few weeks old.

From a purely descriptive point of view, S visited the three areas, one after the other, in a time sequence. These "different visits" coincided with S's different use of her body and mine.

From behaving like a sack of potatoes, completely slumped on the floor or in my arms, S slowly became a "crawling child", who was somehow able to move towards, or away from, the big wardrobe or my body. She entered into these spaces by crawling, or she moved away from them full of anger and disappointment if her omnipotent wishes were frustrated (Area A).

Later, with some determination, S chose to sit on my chair, next to the table with the lamp, but at the same time, in difficult moments, she became quite dependent on my eyes and the upper part of my face. Finally, playing with my glasses, she discovered the difference between her own image, reflected on my lenses and my body, and she also discovered the space that separated us and that between her body and the table. She learned to control this space with her eyes and with her movements in general (Area B). This increased ability to feel in control of herself, her movements and the objects around her, was followed by a growing interest in her body, her mouth, bottom and vagina. Even the table-hand-breast became an object of her primitive exploration, as something separate from her, which sometimes she wanted to control completely and against which, on other occasions, she showed the intensity of her ambivalence (Area C). This evolution in the motor behaviour in the child confirmed the impression that I had about her during our first meeting: at the time, I had thought that her spastic condition was even more serious because of the lack of a genuine curiosity about the external world. S seemed to use her body and movements only to control those of her mother.

The modifications of the emotional experience of S in therapy were accompanied by deep modifications in my own countertransference experience, which greatly helped me to give meaning to her behaviour.

In our very early sessions, when we were still in Area A, my contact with S was hindered by the anxiety that the child might regress at a behavioural level and particularly, that she might lose control over her sphincters or that she might have an epileptic fit. I felt this possible regression as something catastrophic, an unforgivable therapeutic error. The meaning of this fear and its intensity became clearer in the following sessions, when I became aware of the controlling and attacking aspects of S's states of isolation, observing at the same time *to what extent she was in control of those states*. I realised that they were the result of the internal activity of a very seductive and omnipotent force, and this gradually helped me to re-gain a more free position and to see what

S really needed. In that period, the child responded to any kind of discomfort in an undifferentiated manner, as is it were hunger, and not jealousy, fear of being left or being invaded or penetrated by my voice.

My main function therefore was to help her differentiate the various sources of her discomfort, whether internal or external, physical or emotional, like the noises that were coming from outside or inside her body, and to resist her attacks which were mainly linked to her intolerance to any kind of waiting or any response to her requests which might be different from real food and physical contact.

In the second movement inside the therapy room, the need to control the primary object became much more explicit in the transference in the game of the "great big lady". At that point, I became the container of the projection of her baby part and of all the negative feelings that she had experienced in relation to a maternal object felt as demanding and rejecting at the same time. Indeed, the child's primary feeding relationship had been joyless, and later the mother had taken up the role of a teacher. However, my experience with S in this period was not invaded only by feelings of rejection or exclusion, but also by something much subtler which affected my curiosity and my wish to know her. My normal curiosity was gradually replaced by a form of mental control of the situation, similar to what could be created artificially by means of a video recorder. I began to notice that, at the end of every session, I could easily and apparently with great precision, recall the material of the therapy. At the same time, I noticed that this did not lead either to a better understanding of the phenomena I observed, or to a greater emotional involvement. My interest and my receptivity towards the child were interfered by a mental activity of an automatic kind, which made me think of the detailed observations of the mother on S's behaviour, or of how the child mechanically repeated the words and the teachings from his mother in the evening, emptying them of any emotional meaning. It was as if in both situations the joy and the wish to understand each other were replaced by a sterile and controlling recording of mutual behaviours. *In the same way, in the transference the child was controlling me from her "great big lady's throne" and I controlled her with my mental video recorder*. I thought that our similar experience of exclusion was responsible for this degeneration: S might feel desperately excluded from my world just as I might feel excluded from hers. The interpretation of these very painful and primitive feelings led to a few changes.

The third movement was very difficult and painful. S appeared very vulnerable and she easily relapsed in physical activities, although not completely isolated from me. *Giving up her full position as a "great big lady" shed an even more dramatic light on her developmental delay.* I began to feel that she was in trouble, especially at the beginning and at the end of each session, when she was handed over from one adult to the other, lost in the therapy room, surrounded by objects that were too numerous and incomprehensible for her. My function therefore was to contain this new experience of the child: I slowed down every single action and reduced every interpretative therapeutic intervention to its basics. I started to talk only about those objects in the room and those parts of my body and hers, which might have an emotional meaning for our relationship. *Her getting lost among those objects was very dangerous because it was accompanied by the loss of any anchorage to an emotionally significant object.* The ease with which she moved "far away" from me and the very few important things in our shared experience and the difficulty to recall them were an indication of how precarious was her attachment to a good internal breast. Her behaviour in difficult moments reminded me of that of a baby who loses the nipple or the attention of his mother and behaves like a baby in utero.

Final observations

The clinical material seems to suggest that S's main problem was her inability (impossibility) to experience herself as a child external and independent from her primary maternal object. Most of the time, S lived in a state of fusion and confusion with her internal and external object. Her world was still the inside of her mother's body, mainly her breast-womb and her mind, where she felt that food and knowledge were being kept hidden from her. She found it unbearable to live outside mother's internal spaces: she felt expelled in a world she could not understand and, at the same time, she was overwhelmed by a feeling of persecution which came both from inside (her hunger, and the painful noises of her stomach) and outside (the noises from the street, the child who was crying outside and all the unknown things about therapy, including, sometimes, her own therapist). In such moments, she seemed incapable of understanding her experiences, of separating her physical pains from other painful stimuli coming from outside and from a more complex mental reality. Her body, her mind, and that portion of the external world in touch with them were still completely fused together. Under the pressure of what she felt as a massive attack from all sides, the child collapsed and lost her physical balance, which was already very unstable. She became more and more *disintegrated* and *disorganised*, also at a muscular level. It was as if a destructive force devastated her mind and body and that there was no way to contain her either physically or emotionally. After the storm, she appeared very tired and confused. This sequence of events more than once made me think of her premature birth and of her early days of life.

As we have seen, S had different ways of defending herself from this intolerable experience: sometimes she played on the floor all crumpled up like a foetus, completely isolated from all external reality, whereas other times she, in her fantasy, took possession of her maternal object and its contents. This second manoeuvre was probably reinforced by the fantasy of a rich mother who expelled her and took away her food to give it to her other children and to her own internal father or paternal penis. On this regard, I was always struck by the emphasis of the child on food, which showed her interest in the upper part of her mother's body, particularly her breast. It was surprising to see how S was always hungry, always in search of food, of something with which to fill her mouth and stomach. Her stubbornness in trying to find out where I was hiding my best food for the other children was quite remarkable, particularly if compared to her general lack of curiosity. Later, I noticed the same determination in her wish to play with the Yellow Pages book which at a certain level represented the book of knowledge, the unknown, much desired world of the mind of her mother and her therapist.

So far, I have described the internal world of S as I could observe it in the therapy room and feel it in the transference. Her everyday experience with her mother, instead, seemed to be crystallised in a relationship full of orders and commands. In the presence of her mother, S became very controlling, using her in a mechanical, negative, and ungrateful manner. On the other hand, the mother tended to interpret her daughter's behaviours always in terms of "badness and stupidity". Certainly, a vicious circle of mutual misunderstanding had originated between them. It could be said that S no longer believed she could ask her primary object to contain and give meaning to her primitive experience of terror, disintegration and death. This happened mainly because of the depression of the mother, who felt persecuted ("shocked"), by such a damaged daughter. Although S's mother looked after her child a great deal, her capacity to keep a space in her mind in which to receive and transform her daughter's projective and adhesive identification was minimal.

Final discussion

At this point, I think it is important to wonder whether the clinical case of S may add something to our understanding of pervasive developmental disorders; we have taken up this challenge by drawing on Meltzer's idea that "an imaginative use of the Kleinian notion of part-object relation and of the Bionian notion of an alpha function in reverse may allow us to interpret autistic material as one would interpret dreams".

In the final discussion of the previous clinical case, I have written that Thomas' problem was to be unable to transform "his deaf and dumb body into live wood" and at the same time to be acknowledged through his gestures, postures, and movements by his parents' minds as a real child and not as a wooden puppet. I have stated that the biggest obstacle to the development of his personality was linked to an almost total lack of differentiation between the objects of the external and internal world.

In the clinical material of this chapter instead, we see a child who, although showing in some circumstances—like in the early consultation sessions—some behaviours that are similar to T's, has a "talking body" which contains and expresses recognisable emotional sensations and experiences, but that unfortunately does not have an audience that can listen and with which it is possible to interact. Only rarely is S able to find in the physical and mental landscape of her objects a pattern that can help her "find or retrieve herself". One could say that the normal flow of the projective and introjective processes within her object relations seems to be seriously hindered by identity processes of a mimetic kind (of a mainly two-dimensional or obsessive nature) and by "no entry" defences which are typical of the mental functioning of anorexic patients (Polacco, 2003).

At this point our task is to try to understand what is so particular about these identifications in S's personality and to compare them with the physiology of early object relations in early development. We could ask ourselves: in which way does the child assimilate the flow of internal and external experiences in which she is immersed?

In which way does she try to get hold of objects and people outside herself in three-dimensional space? How does she manage their presence or absence in her memory?

To answer these questions, I would suggest we should reflect on three episodes in the therapeutic pathway of the child: I am referring to her slow walk in the area of the soft chair and the doll's house, her discovery of the therapist's face in the "great big lady" game and her activities with hands and mouth in the children's area.

For years, these experiences have uselessly haunted my mind as I searched for an interpretative hypothesis, which might fully reveal their transference and developmental meaning, like dream images that I was unable to forget. From the very beginning, I thought that they might somehow be linked to introjective processes and personal memory, without being able, however, to understand what were the specific mechanisms that regulated them. Later, reading *Live Company* (Alvarez, 1992), I realised, just as Alvarez explains in the following quotation, that my difficulty was due to the fact that the alimentary model, which had always offered helpful metaphors to interpret transference relationships to part objects could not find its realisation in the three experiences mentioned above.

> The alimentary model has offered a rich source of metaphor, for the ways in which experience is assimilated, but it nevertheless needs no longer be the only one. Indeed, when the problem has to do with the patient's difficulties in listening, the breast-mouth model may be inadequate. The manner in which experience is assimilated through the visual modality, and also through tactile modes other than oral ones, (e.g. the ways in which babies improve upon their capacity to reach and grasp objects in three dimensional space) may also provide a fertile source for both theory and technique with psychotic children. The face, for example, that an experience can be assimilated only when it is located in someone else may have more to do with questions of perspective, than with questions of projection. Such locating may actually involve the beginnings of an introjective process rather than a projective one. The way in which a patient may or may not be able to follow his therapist's train of thought, or pursue one of his own, may be as analogous to the problem of the visual tracking of the trajectory of moving objects as to his response to the flow of milk in his throat (Alvarez, 1992, p. 79).

Even the theory of misconception and disorientations suggested by Money-Kyrle (1968), in his paper "The cognitive development", that contains the idea that "the two mental tasks any new born animal has to perform if it is to survive [are] the acquisition of a few, I believe innately predetermined, concepts (or class of notions), and, what is not innately predetermined, the location of their members in a space-time system" (Money-Kyrle, 1968, pp. 417–418), did not envisage that there might be ways different from those suggested by the alimentary experience with which the new born could reach this objective.

Only W. R. Bion ("The imaginary twin", 1950), after observing that his patients who had serious difficulties in personifying the split-off parts of their personality "*seemed to have similar problems that obtruded themselves almost as if concerned with vision itself*" (Bion, 1950, p. 20), had highlighted the importance of sight in the exploration of the environment. Moreover, in his conclusions, he had suggested the possibility that there might be simultaneity between psychological and physical development in the early months of a child's life: "I have wondered whether the psychological development was bound up with the development of ocular control in the same way that problems of development linked with oral aggression co-exist with the eruption of teeth" (Bion, 1950, p. 22).

In the case of S, we see a child who, in her relationship with reality, uses sight and touch as her favourite modalities: this happens because *oral experiences, despite their central role, have a quality which is so anorexic-bulimic that cannot become the metaphor of a link*; they cannot provide the child with the idea of a link that may favour symbolic transformation and development. On the contrary, *they are used to create a situation of "no entry" or of destruction of the object*. As her mother says, S becomes "crazy" when she is hungry or when she feels pains and discomfort in her belly, which she mistakes for hunger. She immediately wants something to put in her mouth, but when she gets what she wants, she often throws it away. The hunger and the pain from her stomach/belly/muscles and skeleton are so full of anxiety and of a sense of death that they must be erased. Other times, when the tongue and the saliva in her mouth seem to saturate every feeling of emptiness and fear, the link with the object is searched for by means of tactile modalities such as stroking, tapping, and skin to skin contact. Also T was very busy "playing" with his hands, tongue, saliva, and mouth: we observe however that the mouth of both children never becomes a stage for sufficiently clear experiences, in a way that what comes in is different from what goes out, what is outside is distinct from what is already inside, what belongs to their body is different from what belongs to the body of their objects. The mouth never becomes a third area, where the double impulse of both children to transform reality and recreate it in their fantasy can be realised.

All this makes one think of the experience of prematurity (S) or of some postnatal physiological immaturity (T) which allowed the children to be aware of the existence of a human object present in their lives only through gazes, caresses, voices in a discontinuous manner, while their oral experience of feeding was either too painfully intrusive or too passive.

We know that in normal development, the breast-fed child does not only feel nourished but also held and thought by the mother.

The oral and aesthetic experiences are intertwined at various levels. But what happens to children like T and S, whose oral experiences are disjointed from tactile, visual, and auditory experiences, when the former are not supported by the latter and vice versa? I think that, in the first case, oral modalities remained primitive and urgent (like the first time that the child is attached to the breast/nipple in the delivery room), whereas in the second case, tactile, visual, and auditory modalities acquired mimetic and superficial or idiosyncratic characters.

I ask myself why a child like S, who could not build a positive model to interpret the flow of experiences through the oral breastfeeding experience, may produce a form of learning from experience that does not stand the test of time, as one can notice in her difficulty to remember the important objects in the room.

What is the meaning of the child's interest in faces?

Is there a difference between locating and picturing a face in space and introjecting it? Must the child perhaps base her idea of a relationship on a virtual experience (visual and tactile modalities in isolation) and not on a real consensual experience? Is then virtual learning preferred to one that is physically experienced? Does this apply only to the child or also to her mother and her therapist?

The feeding experience does not offer to either child an interpretative model of the flow of intersubjective experiences and of reality in motion. Also the therapeutic experience is extraneous to this model, even if it is built on it. Are these perhaps the reasons why the transference movements of patients suffering from pervasive developmental disorders look so different from those of normal patients? It still needs to be understood if and how introjective processes based on exclusively tactile or visual superficial modalities of assimilation of the flow of experiences may consolidate in the psychic reality of the patients. We will attempt to answer this question in the next chapter looking at the clinical material of Rebecca, a psychotic pubertal child.

CHAPTER EIGHT

Rebecca (Re), the child kissed by the Snow Queen: lifeline and perspective as symbolic forms

Introduction

In the previous two chapters I have tried to illustrate the ways in which two children, Thomas and Suzanne, suffering from pervasive developmental disorder, related to the "life experiences" in which they were immersed and which pressed on their physiological and psychic apparatus in order to be taken in and organised with some sense or meaning. Applying the notions of part object and reversed alpha function to the clinical material, I reached the conclusion that there was something wrong in the anatomy and physiology (Caccia, 2012) of their early internal object relations which, in the course of their development, had prevented *their "body" from becoming the metaphor of a human link, and their "mind" from becoming incarnate in their "living body"*.

To this regard, I have pointed out how both children, the first because of the trauma of his neonatal asphyxia and the second because of her premature birth, have entered life in a painful way and in an emotionally deprived context. I have also shown how their developmental delay and their states of isolation within the analytic relationship, although roughly comparable to those of a normal baby in his last months of foetal life and the first months of neonatal life, never appear as preparatory for a new phase of development and expression of those unconscious conflicts and persecutory anxiety and confusional states which can be observed in early infancy.

In this chapter, I will revisit these concepts by analysing some excerpts taken from the clinical material of a psychotherapeutic experience, which lasted a little more than three years, three times a week with a ten-year-old psychotic girl called Rebecca. Here, too, we will observe the same adhesive, imitative modalities of dealing with the "flow" of experiences that we have observed in the clinical material of T and S, but also their "evolution and overcoming". It will therefore be possible to follow what made this achievement possible.

We will see how Re, after months of therapy, was able to use plasticine to create a sculpture, a three dimensional artistic copy of my face and body, and to feel, after regaining her confidence in the goodness of my eyes, that she could express and communicate through her "body" a state of primitive anxiety which for many years had not found a symbolic form inside her. It will be interesting to follow her path towards the discovery of three-dimensionality which was achieved through experiences guided by an intense and curious gaze on me which, from a distance, gathered every details of my face (see S) and body which she then tried to faithfully reproduce by moving and pressing her hands on the material (and therefore with visual and tactile modalities similar to those of T and S). The result of this work was helpful to assess whether the object-therapist had been seen properly in its true characteristics, consequently showing the she had acquired a new capacity to regulate the (emotional) "distance" of her interest on me through a good identification with my way of looking at her.

Finally, we will try to understand whether the clinical material about this patient may provide new evidence to Meltzer's idea that "autism is not a thought disorder but one of its variants" and help us to investigate the reasons why the virtual world of cartoons and films has such a great importance in the construction of the claustrum of these children, and to better understand how we can favour the evolution of their personality starting from their somehow idiosyncratic interests and attitudes towards life.

Case history

When Re started her psychoanalytic psychotherapy, she was just over the age of ten. She had always been a difficult child and in her early infancy had shown a serious delay in her motor development and in her language, so that from the age of three and a half, she had been looked after in a private structure for autistic children. In the last weeks before our first meetings, on the occasion of a visit to the town zoo, Re had started behaving in a "crazy" way. At school, she had pooed and peed in her pants on more than one occasion and she had started playing with her excrements. During religious ceremonies in the synagogue, she had behaved in a very provocative manner, showing her genitals to the people who came close to her, attacking them with different types of vulgar expressions. At home, she had spent long periods of time masturbating, accompanying this activity with triumphant laughter and noisy incomprehensible soliloquies. Teachers and parents had also noticed that the child sometimes left this world of anal and genital excitement but only to withdraw and isolate herself in a deep mutism, sitting by herself for a long time, motionless on a chair or on her bed, with one thumb deep in her throat and hiding her face with the other hand. In her excited state, she did not seem in touch with her mental or physical suffering, or with the hostility that her behaviour caused in other people. In her state of isolation, she seemed to be overwhelmed by something intolerable. Re came from a poor family who lived in a working-class area. The parents also had another daughter, two years her senior. The mother, a very ailing person, was the only one to accept to take the child to the clinic three times a week, fulfilling her commitment regularly until the end. I never had the opportunity to meet her personally because she was seen by a psychiatric social worker once a week. Her GP told me that she had suffered from eclampsia during her pregnancy and of a deep depression after the birth of her child, while Re had had a very painful breastfeeding experience in her first weeks of life because of an oral thrush. The father, who never actively took part in her daughter's psychotherapeutic experience and whom I never met, lived at home and had a manual job there.

The first period of therapy: "an amusing mind"

The first time I met Re I was struck by the expressive intensity of her movements, her posture and her way of exploring the space around her with her eyes. At first, the child came towards me hopping and flapping her arms like wings, without looking at me. In her left hand she held a flat handbag, from which the pointed face of a soft toy emerged. She was a prepubescent child, rather chubby and short. As I walked with her along the corridor towards the therapy room, she began to shuffle her feet on the floor, as if they were made of lead. I then noticed that she was very badly dressed, there were holes in her socks and in her jumper, and the skin of her face was greasy and dirty. She looked like a sick, mentally insufficient girl. In contrast with all this, her eyes were dark, bright and mobile. Once in the room, with a "grand lady" attitude, she thoroughly inspected the therapy room, immediately complaining about its poor furniture, showing her great skill in grasping at a glance the singularities of the new situation in which she had found herself. After this critical remark, naturally made without addressing me directly, she moved towards the table, showing her interest in the toy box that I had prepared for her. As soon as she opened the lid of the box, she immediately put her handbag on the window ledge, grabbed the plasticine and quickly and skilfully she shaped a multi-coloured elephant with a pointy hat. Then, she began punching holes in its body using the legs of a little horse. She asked me if I was a doctor who treated children with measles. Without giving me the time to answer her question, she added that she had come to the clinic because she had the measles. After a brief pause, she burst into laughter, raised her eyes towards me without looking at me, and told me that she had come to see me because her mind was "funny and amusing". Then, forgetting about me, she went on punching holes in the elephant's body, calling it monster and giggling to herself.

A grand overture.

The "star system" of the clinic

In the following sessions, Re began to let me understand what she thought about the clinic and the people that she met in the waiting room. She transformed her work desk into the stage of a theatre on which she performed different stories with characters that she herself made out of plasticine. Occasionally, she paused to draw the same stories, with the same characters, on sheets of paper or on the walls of the room. As if fishing them out of a magical top hat, she staged a crowd of characters, monsters and witches, jugglers and lion tamers from a circus, pets and wild animals. These characters performed various acts of cruelty, stole, killed, and made dangerous acrobatics, always in front of a human or animal baby, who was the passive witness of these acts of violence. "The monster-elephant with the measles" also took part in these performances, turning into a gunman, an armoured soldier, a strong muscular man, a skilful juggler, a cold lion tamer, a great dancer according to the scene, but always in the role of the main character, the protagonist, the winner. Seduced by this very powerful figure, able to prevail in a ruthless world populated by magicians, witches, evil men and exhibitionist acrobats, Re did not seem to be worried about the danger to which the babies were exposed. Also the female characters in her play, instead of looking after their young, only seemed to be striving to get the alpha male or to get a centre stage position, like the stars of a ballet company. As the end of our session approached, her game became darker. The elephant with the holes turned into an evil, disturbing, and threatening character: a monster with long, sharp teeth, like those of a walrus or with its knees covered with poisonous quills; an Indians with feathers on his hat and with a Chinese-looking pony tail, talking quickly and menacingly; or a female monster with a great belly, on which the image of a baby fox-devil was engraved. On more than one occasion, I tried to stop Re to ask her to explain her game to me, with the only result of seeing her withdraw even more. Clearly persecuted by my words and my presence, she did whatever she could to keep away from me and in order to negate my presence, with quick and skilful gestures, she immediately changed the script and the scene of her story.

It was as if she were holding a magic wand from which a cloud of stardust skilfully emerged, which quickly turned into a new world.

In contrast with this excited activity, however, Re often complained that she was "tired". This mainly happened on the threshold of the therapy room, which we reached after going down a ramp of stairs. She spelt it out as if she wanted to make sure that I listened to her. Also on these occasions she did not look at me and she did not seem to want to talk to me. Indeed, if I showed her that I wanted to get closer and talk about her being tired, Re immediately ran away, towards the table, where she started playing with the bad monsters in an increasingly excited and fast-paced manner, or she walked to the window on the opposite side of the entrance, where she got lost in long, senseless rants, a sort of verbal diarrhoea.

Towards the end of the third week of therapy, a trivial flu prevented Re from coming for three sessions in a row. When she came back, she looked stunned and frightened for what had happened to her. She kept repeating that she had had a fever because of the very cold weather. She constantly touched her forehead to check whether she was still hot. She breathed heavily, as if she was not certain she was well. She was quite restless and showed a constant need to be reassured about her health. She asked me several times to go back to her mother in the waiting room, as if the therapy room had become an infected, suffocating place. In this state of anxiety and confusion, she told me several times that I, too, had been ill. She tried, as was her habit, to stop my words in any way she could for the whole session. Finally, to my great surprise, she calmed down and sat on the table. She opened the toy box and in a determined tone of voice she told me that she did not like the monsters anymore. Immediately after that, she grabbed the plasticine monster-elephant with the measles and resolutely tore it to pieces making it disappear.

I thought at once that during the illness, the fever, the forced rest at home, the absence from school and from therapy, Re had spent most of her time masturbating, and that she had concretely got lost in sexual feelings and fantasies for which she was not prepared, which now frightened her and that she could not get rid of. Her anxiety of being in a hot, suffocating, contaminated place made me think that even the therapy room had become for her a place of erotic pleasure and had turned in her mind, during our separation, into a nuptial chamber or into the genitals of the analytic couple. Destroying the monster elephant with the measles, therefore, could have two meanings: on one hand, she no longer wanted to be seen by me as a baby with the measles; on the other, she no longer trusted me because I had abandoned her to indulge in my own sexual pleasure, which she felt as something dirty and bad which polluted my mind.

After this separation from therapy, Re was no longer the same; she replaced the monster-elephant with something else and her play with some other activities. She started coming to the sessions always bringing with her a colour picture of a man's naked body all covered with long hairs, which she had torn off one of her father's magazines. She kept it on the table or she hung it on the walls of the room watching it for a while. When she was not absorbed in this activity, she went on exploring every corner of the room, complaining that it was too hot. She constantly touched her forehead, peeled off the dead skin from her face and she became absorbed as she played with the hairs of her own legs.

As darkness approached, she often stopped to see her reflection in the window—panes, where she could see both her face and mine. She danced excitedly in front of the window, or she moved the table next to window ledge, lay on it, face down, and started to touch her genitals. She was unreachable, and she spoke loudly in an incomprehensible fragmented language, interrupted by malicious laughter. She often said "vagina" as she touched her genitals, and she laughed like a witch. Sometimes she wetted her fingers with her own sweat or vaginal secretions and used them to write on the window pane, or on the surface of the table, tracing letters or drawing mysterious pictures.

Only on one occasion, at the beginning of a session, did she change her attitude for a second: she stopped on the threshold of the playroom and excitedly, without looking at me, she said that when "she was little she had hated walking". I remembered that when she was younger she had started walking very late, and that her first steps had been those of a ballerina.

I asked her if when she told me about her childhood experience she wanted to talk to me about something that also had to do with some of her current experiences, her sexuality in particular.

But I was left thinking that perhaps Re was telling me that she hated to come to therapy, just as she had hated walking as a young child, because she felt that something was beyond her control. I thought that she had experienced her illness as a "ruinous fall" which had suddenly interrupted her first steps in therapy, putting her in touch with something intolerable, which she now tried to control and digest in her sessions.

Later, on the occasion of her first period, she told me that she hated all new things, or those, which happen to her too soon. "I hate early things": she told me.

Commentary

With these notes, I hope I have succeeded in providing a sufficiently clear idea of the type of experience to which I was exposed in my therapeutic work with Re. It is this precisely in these initial moments of the therapy with psychotic children that the therapist meets the greatest difficulties in putting together their material in an attractive as well meaningful way, in order to reach them and attract their attention towards him, in an attempt to save them from their folly.

From the clinical material, it is evident that Re seemed to have lost any hope of being understood. She was no longer able to make herself known and express something about her real Self. On one hand, she was imprisoned by her excited activity, which removed from her play activity, her representations and identifications any depth and communicative value; she found herself in a totally solipsistic position, which made her feel "up to the situation", making her feel totally in control. On the other hand, she plunged into states of silent retreat. When a sudden, unexpected event like her illness took her out of her manic position, she seemed to get in touch with an intolerable experience, like a "ruinous" fall from which she recovered finding shelter, once again, in her world of mental excitement (the amusing mind) or sexual excitement (her vagina). What most struck me when I observed Re's behaviour was the paroxysm, which characterised both her manic position and her reaction to an experience of anxiety; this removed all emotional meaning from her link with me and with reality. This made me think that in Re's internal world, in her deep intersubjective communications, something was lacking: an essential human quality which might help her feel contained in her omnipotence and supported in her despair.

At the same time, carefully exploring my interpretative activity, I could observe my difficulty in finding words, images, which might be communicable and interesting to the child. I too felt imprisoned within a solipsistic position. When I was busy organising Re's play in my mind, considering the fundamental moments of the session—approach, presence, and separation—according to the theoretical model which associates the analytical experience to the primary relationship of the child with the maternal object, I became aware that my communications, although intellectually fulfilling and in many aspects supported by clear evidence, did not meet any emotional response from the child. On the other hand, the moment when Re confronted me with her depression and fear, on the threshold of the room, I felt incapable of finding in my mind something that might give shape to what I was experiencing and which might reverberate and amplify the child's experiences.

To use a part-object metaphor, I noticed that my interpretative activity, as well as my attention and my gaze, became for the mind-mouth of the child a kind of thought-nipple whose tone, in certain moments, was not strong enough to be grasped and, in other moments, too hard to be accepted. For example, I was overwhelmed by the great wish to sleep in the first case, or I tended to become chatty and intrusive in the second. It seemed to me, therefore, that the compositional quality which I could not translate in my communications, had to do with the ability of a mother to explore and compose the experience of her child with "the right tone" (Bertolini, 1998).

The second period of therapy: the crazy hats

Immediately after her return from the summer holidays, a year after the beginning of therapy, Re greeted me and said: "Don't you see that

I have grown up? I am no longer interested in monsters, animals, and ballerinas; I only think about punks, skinheads, and disco dancers."

She was taller and thinner, and she had cut her hair short. From then on, Re started coming to session wearing strange little hats, called "crazy hats", with long antennae, on top of which were attached stars, dice, and miniature spirals of different colours. Her general attitude towards therapy became increasingly contemptuous. At first she attacked the rules of the therapeutic setting: more than once she refused to come to the room on time, put up some resistance when it was the end of her session, started throwing her toys out of the window and made several attempts to get out of the room to go to the toilet without my permission or to intrude into other rooms in the clinic.

Then she changed her strategy, and began to attack more directly my ability to think. After a particularly long weekend, because of a national bank holiday that fell on a Monday:

> She arrived in therapy with a very bizarre object: a horse's head stuck into a plastic bottle. At first, she put it between her legs, to masturbate. Then she detached the horse's head and threw it away, in a corner of the room, and sticking the bottle in her mouth as if it were a trumpet, she started walking around the room excitedly, pretending to play the music of Coronation Street, a popular British TV programme.

A few weeks later, on a Monday:

> She arrived in a quite excited state. Without even giving me the time to say hello, she started telling me three Jewish stories (we had three weekly sessions) that I did not know, and she went on talking non-stop for more than half an hour. She told me all three of them simultaneously, so that the theme of one story intersected and overlapped those of the other two, and vice versa, causing a great confusion on a verbal level. At the same time, the story was also punctuated by sudden pauses and interruptions, during which Re lost the thread of her narrative. She always reacted to these gaps with panic, at first, and then with a big, triumphant laughter, after which she carried on with her story, adding some other absolutely incomprehensible details, which complicated her already intricate plots even further. The final result was that of a great confusion which left very little space for thinking.

On this occasion I was struck by the look of panic that Re showed every time she lost the thread of her narrative, and by her compulsive need to fill in all her memory lapses with fragments from another story. The child's speech behaviour was the same as her walking behaviour when she was little; it was something similar to Antonio's experience with his bicycle (see Chapter Four): in the area of knowledge and language, I could observe the equivalent of her "walking on tiptoe like a ballerina" when she was little, as if the important moments of developmental change triggered in her a hatred for any type of dependence and frustration.

At the same time, she did not seem aware that the gaps in her narrative depended on her belief that she knew everything at once and very well (her omniscience), just as she had not been aware that part of her falls, when she had started walking, had not been the consequence of her lack of experience, but of her stubborn impulse to walk on tiptoe.

In both situations, she associated her failures to something dangerous and humiliating, as if a malevolent person had attacked her from the outside or had wanted to play a dirty trick on her. Re was unable to differentiate the mental state of being in intrusive identification from that of being out of it, and to keep both of them in her mind at the same time, as two different viewpoints on her experience. Instead, she felt that with her pauses, the discontinuity of her narrative and her mistakes, she could easily become the potential target for the destructive criticism of an internal or external observer. Even more so, she could not grasp in the gaps the evidence of her false grandiosity. She was instead helplessly witnessing the transformation of the wonderful view she had of herself, of the marvellous dress she thought she was wearing, into a net full of holes, which tightened around her to the point of suffocation.

The prison of intrusive identification

At this point, I believe it is important to stop and think about the quality of Re's personifications with the monster-elephant with the pointy hat and holes on its skin, with the hairy man of the photograph from the magazine, and with the punk girl with coloured visors and magical antennae. In the first identification, Re seems to be confused with a disturbing character because of its badness and urge to be at the centre of attention. In the second, she seems lost within an erotised object, warm but suffocating; and in the third she is identified with a magical mind which controls every thought (Re becomes the mistress of the three compartments of the maternal body: anus, genitals, breast-mind).

These personifications absorb a great part of the child's attention, guiding and orienting her behaviour in the session, supporting her sense of identity and pushing her into a state of isolation. In all three situations, Re seems to own identifications which make her "feel up to it", which give her "a tone"; she seems to want to pursue her interests in the same way she had tried to walk: on tiptoe like a ballerina even before making her real first steps. All this happens in such a paroxystic way, quick and exhibited, that these identifications are flattened and devoid of any complexity. What she shows to her therapist does not establish nor support an emotional link. It attracts the therapist's attention, but makes it impossible—or particularly difficult to him—to get access to the feelings and emotions that are activated by the analytic relationship. There is something in her way of getting hold of reality and exhibit it that makes her emotion or her initial feeling unknowable, preventing both the child and the therapist from learning and truly experiencing it.

What strikes in Re is particularly her way of talking, which brings to the mind the image of a skin affected by the measles: her verbal language, just like a diseased skin, is full of gaps, like the steps of a dancer and of startling, sudden events, like her laughter or her memory lapses.

The face and eyes of the therapist: the first introjective processes

Alongside this state of things, which seemed to establish either a negative therapeutic reaction or a situation of persecutory depression with hypochondriac connotations, without hope (the phenomenology of intrusive identification), from the first year of therapy, there began to be moments in which Re appeared genuinely curious about me, showing particular interest in my face and eyes.

As a matter of fact, she sometimes came to sessions wearing red and green visors covering her eyes, through which she stared at me for quite a while. The green and red made me think of a traffic light, of traffic rules and therefore of my paternal functions within the therapeutic context. Other times, she did a similar thing with a red transparent ruler, as if she wanted to measure me up or once again tried to understand the sense of my rules.

On another occasion, she seemed to be able to keep her attention on me for a longer period of time, sharply splitting the upper part of my body from the genital area through a game of alternate gazes, as if she wanted to preserve a good relationship at least with one part of me. She watched me intensely, trying to focus her gaze on me. In particular, she seemed to be looking for something in my eyes or face to hold on to, something which could act as a reference point, a sort of organising focus free from the "special" perspectives of arrogance, excitement, seduction, and self-satisfaction which were the dominant characteristics of her transference in that period.

Another time she stared at me for a long time through some red-coloured filters that she had found in the waiting room. Originally, they were part of a holographic game with coloured blots in a book, which became three-dimensional and clear if observed through them.

These games made me think that at this point of the therapeutic process there was the possibility for a new type of research, which had to do with introjective processes. For the first time Re showed that she was able to leave the paroxysm of her fantasies of omnipotence and impotence, and she became genuinely interested in my eyes, as if she had wanted to explore the meaning of my attentive gaze on her. Staring at my eyes for a long time, without telling me anything about what was on her mind, it seemed as if she wondered whether they were a dangerous appendix of my body, like my genitals, or equally dangerous holes. Just as the slightly swollen spots of the measles, were confused with the holes she had made in the skin of the monster-elephant, my eyes began to be perceived as an emergence in the background which in her mind was confused with a sort of discontinuity, as something real, but seen from an excessive distance. In this way, Re helped me to understand how difficult it was for her to find the right distance to look at me (and be looked at by me) within the analytic relationship, showing that something was damaged in her conception of the primary object.

Negative contagion and falling like a rag doll

In the period after the first summer holiday, on more than one occasion, I began to experience moments of sudden drowsiness. Unexpectedly, above all in the course or at the end of an interpretation, I plunged, against my will, into a dreamless sleep. I did not lose the thread of my argument or the interest in what I was saying because the child was not listening to me, however. In fact, I did not even have the time to feel inadequate or angry: the thread of my attention had already broken.

My words were emptied of meaning and disappeared in a void without leaving any trace, just like soap bubbles in the air. For a moment I thought that I had fallen ill, and that my drowsiness was due to fits of narcolepsy. For the first time in my life I was experiencing a sort of discontinuity unrelated to any physical sensation and devoid of emotional meaning. I linked my drowsiness to the experience of Re when she found herself emptied in her head, with a black hole left by the broken thread of the narrative during the telling of the three stories. I associated all this to what she had told me several times before, about her intolerance towards the end of the sessions and all the unpredictable and uncontrollable events in her life (her high fever, the sudden thunderstorm). There was something terrifying in unplanned events which made her react in a manic way, destroying the awareness of time, becoming confused, absurdly and tenaciously holding on to known events (the seasons, the colours in the room or of my face), which were distant from the turbulence of emotions.

In any case, I felt that these experiences of loss of control in my attention had occurred precisely because a deep contact with Re had somehow been established; therefore, a negative phenomenon became visible just because it was rooted in a process that was charged with interest; thus I felt encouraged to believe that I was following the right path. All these reflections led me to try to consolidate and protect all the aspects of R's personality, which were attracted by the kind of work we were doing. This effort made it possible for Re to experience something similar to what I have just described and, in particular, to feel that she should neither be frightened nor get excited if something happened that might painfully interfere with her life experiences.

A few weeks later:

Re came to her session wearing a Mickey Mouse T-shirt.

She had spent a quiet weekend at home with her family. In the room, she took out two kangaroos from her box, a young, thin one, and a fat, adult one. She started making them jump on the table. I tried to ask her something about these two kangaroos, and she replied, rather confusedly, saying something about the TV programme Coronation Street, which reminded me of her orgy with the trumpet. Then she set the two kangaroos aside and started working on a piece of plasticine. Carefully looking at me more than once and for quite some time, she shaped a human figure. After finishing it, she started to empty it from the inside, the body and the head in particular, as if she were preparing a plaster cast in which to pour molten bronze in

> order to make a statue. Then she repeatedly tried to make it stand, without success. I told her that perhaps there were very intense feelings in her which led her, secretly and greedily, to get hold of my contents, ending up in the company of a doctor who could not stand on his feet, having been emptied from the inside. At this point Re grabbed another piece of plasticine, and very quickly shaped another character: a girl with ice-skates. She then started to make her skate on the table and in the air. I told her that she was that child: in order not to feel empty she started to run and skate magically. Thinking of the icy surface, I reminded her that our time was almost over. Then, Re took another piece of plasticine and shaped it into a long salami roll, which she cut in many little pieces, as if they were toffee, and she pretended to eat a few. Then she shaped another piece of plasticine into a cigar, which she pretended to smoke. I talked to her about her wish to be "tough" like a male, playing on the assonance "toffee"/"tough", and to be able to feel that she did not need me.

After this session, Re spent more and more time, in the middle part of our sessions, trying to shape the figure of her therapist with plasticine and to empty it from the inside. I did not fully understand the meaning of her insistence in wanting to empty the statuette from the inside, even if it became clearer, as time went by, that her worries were focused on the theme of my absences, which seemed to trigger in the child feelings of greed (emptying the statuette) and of homicidal jealousy.

One Wednesday, shortly before a seven-day break:

> Re's mother approached me in the waiting room to tell me that her child had been rather shocked by a piece of news that she had read in the local papers: four children had been burned to death in house fire. I did not talk to her about it straight away, but she herself told me about it in the course of a session.
>
> As soon as she saw me in the waiting room, Re said "No, no", to make it clear that she did not want to come into the therapy room with me. After a few minutes she stood up from her chair and started following me. In her right hand she was holding an apple with three holes from which she had greedily sucked all its contents. She asked me why I was wearing a pair of jeans and not my usual blue suit, which in her eyes was the clinic's uniform. I replied that these changes in me made her feel very suspicious, and maybe today she could not experience me as good and therefore to trust me. In the room, I asked her something about the three holes in her apple, and I suggested she should think about the approaching analytic holidays and

about the three sessions that would be cancelled. She did not reply, but made a gesture with her hand as if wanting to squeeze me, empty me like her apple.

Then she opened the toy box and split all the animals in two groups. On one side she placed the ox and the cow, and on the other all the other animals in a row, ready to play rounders.

Unlike other times, she did not start playing at once, but she told me that the three holes in her apple also stood for the three O's of ZOO 50, a badge from London Zoo, and she remembered of her visit to the London Zoo; she had returned home quite excited and confused after seeing some animals mating and some birds exhibit their plumage in order to attract their sexual partners. After a pause she added that she wanted to talk to me about her breasts and of how she would soon have to wear a bra. She burst into laughter, looking both sly and seductive. I replied that maybe inside her there was a struggle between a part of her that wanted to protect her breasts, and another part that, instead, would have liked to show them to me, just like the birds' plumage, selling them cheaply as she had done in the past with her genitals, her bottom and her mouth.

In this conflict I could perceive her attempt to protect the therapy from her infantile envy and greed, which she had enacted by emptying the apple that represented a good relationship with the therapy-breasts. I pointed out to her how her excitement took away all meaning from her relationship with me, and how she had partly tried to empty my words of their meaning, which invited her to think of her feelings about our imminent separation.

After this interpretation, Re calmed down, and for a while she seemed to be absorbed in her own thoughts; then she "woke up" and she furiously threw all the animals on the floor, telling me that something was crying in her mind. After several attempts, she managed to tell me that this crying had to do with the four children who had died in the fire. She stood up from her chair and with court-like vehemence she started telling me that the au-pair girl was to blame for the death of the children: she had come home drunk, and she had dropped the candle that had set the house on fire. She also added that the baby in the cradle had survived, because he had managed to climb over the sidebars and to escape from the fire all by himself.

I pointed out that she had thrown all the animals off the table, as if they stood for the dead, crying children whom she now felt inside herself. Maybe she felt that something was at risk of death also inside her every time she masturbated and became "hot", as if she herself were burning something or someone inside her body. These children, perhaps, whom she attacked in her mind, stood for my other patients or my own children, of whom she was

> very jealous, and therefore she could no longer love them or look after them in herself, becoming towards them a bit like a drunk and murderous baby sitter. I added that she was perhaps telling me that she could also, sometimes, feel abandoned by me, by a busy mother, in the hands of an evil baby-sitter.
>
> Re picked up the toys from the floor, one by one, and eventually she got ready to play rounders. All the animals were placed in a row, and each one of them had to wait their turn to strike. At this point it seemed as if Re wanted to stage one of her school or sports experiences (maybe more as a spectator than a participant), in which all the children were asked to take part with order and discipline in the rounders game, which is similar to baseball. Re began to throw a plasticine ball towards every animal, which in turn responded trying to strike it with its bat. The one that managed to throw it the farthest was the winner. She played this game several times, getting more and more tired.

Two sessions later, one Monday after the weekend:

> Re came back with some liquorice in her mouth, sucking it very greedily and ostentatiously. She sat down next to the table and started playing rounders with the animals. She was very withdrawn and distant, engrossed in her activities, when she unexpectedly lost control of her head, which fell forward, violently hitting her chin against her chest, as if she suddenly fallen asleep. She recovered at once and, quite frightened, remarked loudly that her head was "floppy". She looked outside the window, and then she told me that a germ had got into her head and had made her ill.

It was as if a germ had made a hole in her head and had emptied it, just as she had done before, when she had emptied the breast and body of her mother, or the plasticine copy of her therapist.

These episodes of sudden loss of muscular tone in her neck, of cataplexy, were repeated in the weeks that followed the analytic holiday, alternating with moments when she felt tired and sleepy.

The sudden attacks of drowsiness, which had attracted my attention in the previous months, were now something that Re herself was experiencing. She reacted to these experiences, on one hand, by increasing the violence of her verbal and physical attacks on me, and on the other, by spending most of the time withdrawn in total isolation, touching various parts of her body, carefully observing the grooves of her rubber soles and the size and brand of her shoes, stretching the elastic band of her underwear and let it go again, and sucking her left thumb in complete silence. She seemed to be telling me that she was self-sufficient, and at the same time she was protesting, because the therapy was exposing her to painful experiences, which she hated, just as she had hated walking when she was a young child.

The featureless face and the face of the clown

Meanwhile, the Christmas holidays were approaching, during which I would have to go away for a week, for the second time in the course of her therapy. On learning about my leave, Re started drawing again, this time in a more compulsive manner. This activity seemed to make her feel more secure and integrated, as if she were wrapped inside a psychological second skin. She spent all the time in her sessions, until our separation, drawing continuously. She revised her old drawings, completing them in various parts; she added some colour to those in black and white; she added some new shapes and other patterns. In the end, it was almost impossible to distinguish what she had drawn in the past from what she had added more recently. From all this confusion, which tended to cover the sheets of paper completely, there gradually emerged some frequent images, characters, and personifications that represented different parts of her.

At first, an image appeared, a "super girl" character, with sensual, red lips and straight, wild hair, like the thoughts in Re's mind. This was often represented by an actress, which was excluded from the excitement and fame of the stage, and was therefore cold and evil like the *Snow Queen*. Then Re drew a part of herself as a child, that was soon personified in a game with the toys, where a little girl rode around the room on a wonderful horse or a camel (after filling the space between the two humps with some plasticine), but was easily thrown off when a small kangaroo made its appearance.

Finally, in her drawings, also her alienated part began to emerge, represented by a small female character with a featureless face, which always appeared on the side of a circular skating rink, where a group of children played hockey.

This is the end of the last session before the Christmas break:

> Re opens her box, looking for something to play with, but cannot find what she is looking for because of its big mess, and she becomes angry. So I ask

> her what she is looking for, and she tells me that she wants the camel. I look for it on her behalf, and I give it to her. She grabs it happily, and with a piece of plasticine she immediately fills the hole between the two humps and places the girl character on top. She makes them "stroll" around on the table, but then she suddenly the little kangaroo makes its appearance, bossily throwing the little girl off the camel's back, replacing her with the father character. Holding the girl character in her hand, R tells me that now she has become D., her autistic friend. She places her on the back of a kangaroo that is standing on the back of an ox, so that little D. reaches the same height as the daddy character sitting on top of the camel, and she starts fighting against him, to unsaddle him. As a weapon, she uses a piece of the fence. In the midst of this clash, the baby character also arrives, climbs beside the girl D., does a couple of somersaults on the fence and then leaves.
>
> Re takes the mummy-puppet from the box and holds it tight in her hands, as if she wanted to squeeze it, making the same gesture she did with the apple in the past. Then she puts down all the human characters and takes a piece of plasticine instead. She spreads it with the palm of her hand and with the large side of a barrier with three holes, which are used for joining other pieces in order to build fences or enclosures. She presses hard on the surface of the plasticine, so that three bumps come out of the three holes. She looks at them and then, not satisfied, flattens them with her fingers. She grabs a calf, and with one of its legs she makes three cuts on the surface of the plasticine, drawing two eyes and a mouth. She says to me: "I am making the face of a clown".

In the weeks that followed the Christmas break, Re told me that she was no longer afraid of the fire; however, in her mind, she had felt strange since she had cut of the tail of all her toy animals. She often complained that her box, which contained all the material used in therapy, was blue, letting me know that the colour blue made her sad. For this reason, she expressed her wish to paint it in a happier colour, in yellow, like the walls of the room.

A daydream

Regarding this period of the therapy, I would like to talk about a personal experience, a sort of daydream, that I had on the occasion of a visit to a modern art exhibition at the Barbican Centre of London (Aftermath, March 1982). While I was at the far end of a large museum hall, I was attracted by a group of paintings that I was not able to see well, because of their distance from me. One of them, in particular, looked like a dark crack on a white background. I got a little closer to the corner of the room where the works of A. Giacometti were exhibited, and I gradually began to notice that the crack had the outline of a human face: it was the face of the artist's mother. I was struck by the expressive intensity and the sculpture-like of the portrait. A few brush strokes had been enough to create an image full of expression and meaning. At the same time, I became interested in some other sculptures by the same artist, and I noticed how the statues had been shaped by reducing the mass of their matter to the minimum, exalting their expressiveness by means of a peculiar distribution of their bodily volumes and an accurate and original shaping of their bronze surfaces so as to capture endless effects of lights and shadows on the statues.

I associated this experience to my initial attempts to give shape to the analytic experience with Re, as well as to her own attempts to give shape, by means of drawings or plasticine, to something inside herself, her own internal object, or inner experience, which seemed to be characterised by a great sense of emptiness and absence of forms; I wished that she might, sooner or later, find her own "Giacometti" inside herself, who might help her with her expressive efforts. In his *A Concise History of Modern Sculpture* (1964), Herbert Read describes in great detail the nature of the difficulties that one may encounter while exploring the most painful parts of one's personality; talking about the art of Giacometti, he indeed states that:

> Attempts have been made to claim Giacometti for realism in art, or even for humanism, but the human body has for him only the significance of being the outward symbol of an intangible subjectivity. A mournful sense of inner emptiness, which cannot in any physical sense be "filled", may perhaps be redeemed by some solid symbol. But the symbol must not be too solid or precise in contours. (Read, 1964, pp. 159–60)

Otherwise, one might add, Re will flatten it, empty it or uproot it, just as she does with my eyes.

Commentary

In this second period of therapy we can observe the constant efforts of Re to give meaning and shape to her therapeutic experience, and in particular, to the attraction of her therapist's face and eyes on her. Immediately after the summer break, Re shows all her hatred for the therapist and the therapy, defining them useless and stupid. Her "escapes" into an accentuated, almost grotesque, adolescent mimicry (with her disguises) or adult mimicry (like in the telling of the three Jewish stories), reveal her great fear of dependence, which seems to have two distinct sources: on one hand, her painful infantile experience with a depressed, absent and at the same time irritable mother; and on the other, her current experience in therapy, with its human and containing qualities, which makes her feel good and safe, but which also, in certain moments, triggers in her such emotional conflicts, so painful that cannot be thought. Her sense of identity is very often supported by masturbatory activities that give strength to her fantasies of intrusive identification with the internal objects in her mind, and it takes on an almost delusional quality, like in the game of the trumpet-horse. The therapeutic struggle, therefore, primarily consists in clarifying these confusions in her experience of identity and in trying to keep alive the feelings and the anxieties arising in her as she participates in the therapeutic process.

In parallel to this, Re seems to be committed to focusing on the face and eyes of her therapist, finding the right filter, the right wavelength that might help her introject them.

It is not easy for her to make it possible for the light coming from my eyes—if it encounters the right light from hers—to produce a three-dimensional image of our link, just like in a holographic print. In her scrutiny, her dominant need is to control and possess me, to "photograph" and flatten me, or to "steal my eyes and turn them into her magical antennae", rather than to "encounter them" and, through them, feel she can "stay with me". A direct, profound contact with her only lasts a few seconds, and then—as if her attention gave in to the effort and her lens went out of focus—her gaze seems to go beyond my eyes, through them. Looking is replaced by staring, guided by "special perspectives" that nullify the acknowledgement of our link.

At this point, the fundamental therapeutic effort seems to be that of distinguishing, on her behalf, the point of view of the "special perspective" from that of three-dimensionality, and of recreating, with my eyes, a centre of convergence so that her attention can be attracted again, outside her omnipotence and omniscience.

It is indeed because I am engaged in this therapeutic effort that I have experienced sudden lapses of attention, falling into a dark, dreamless sleep. What I experience in such moments feels foreign to my way of being, but it is somehow justified by the child's situation. My sudden drowsiness, as I have said before, occurred in the midst of my interpretative efforts, and it introduced a very painful discontinuity in my experience of identity, foreign to the mental processes that I acknowledge as my own. My deep feeling is that, as I speak, Re does not consciously or unconsciously, oppose my interpretations or the emotional meanings that I try to convey to her with my words, but rather, that she is already elsewhere. In those moments, there is nothing in her that makes her receptive to the contents and the syntax of my words.

These experiences make me think about her panic reactions when she loses the thread of her stories, and I realise that such reactions are not just the expression of her fear of a persecutor that wants to humiliate her because he has found out about her fraudulence and inadequacy, but also of a persecutor who devours her brain, robs her of all her attributes, emptying and flattening her.

In the months that followed, Re begins to experience lapses of attention that are similar to mine, with a loss of control of the muscular tone of her head on her chest, suddenly becoming like a rag doll. She experiences these atonic crises in a very persecutory manner, attributing them to the attack of an outside germ that makes her ill. In a way that is almost symmetrical to my experience, for the first time Re seems to become aware of something that somehow breaks the thread of her attention, thus interrupting an activity that interests her. There is something quite new, however: while, in the past, this experience would have been evacuated with a laugh, or idealised, now that Re is more emotionally involved with me and begins to feel the emotional weight of her separation from the therapy, she feels that the loss of control of her muscular tone is a dangerous phenomenon that clashes with her deepest wishes and interests. These phenomena take place when the task of constructing and protecting her link with me becomes more difficult, like before and after an interruption in the analytic process, and her attention is not supported from within. They seem to belong to her old autistic ways, which were used in the past to avoid any kind of psychic suffering. Now, her interest for our link is so important that her autistic manoeuvre is felt as a dangerous interference, as an illness, in her contact with reality.

The last period of therapy, over the Christmas holidays, shows a positive evolution in Re's efforts to imagine herself and the therapist.

She gradually seems to discover in herself a guide that keeps her oriented towards an object, which attracts her and re-awakens the turbulence of her emotional life. Alongside this, also her infantile parts begin to have a face, revealing different features according to the different emotions that they represent.

The premature end of therapy: a difficult search for identity

The third year of therapy was characterised by three major events, in terms of external reality: the decision—due to external circumstances—to end therapy within a year; the onset of menstruations; and the passage from primary to middle school. Initially, Re reacted to these three big changes with anxiety and moments of powerful regression. Then she quickly started to develop again, showing her surprising willpower.

The main theme was the search for an identity of her own, authentic, truthful, separate from her original objects but in tune with the wish to own the competences and the physical and emotional skills of her peer group.

For a very long period, the main character of her play activity was a small rag dog, named "perfumed puppy", a dirty and broken soft toy that she brought from home and that had belonged to her since she was a baby. She treated it very badly during her sessions, banging it everywhere, throwing it in the air, or even using it to masturbate herself. She also spent long periods of time making "magic hats", which she made the puppy wear. Sometimes she would place the puppy inside one of her red gym shoes, as if it were a wonderful dog basket. She never let the dog lie calmly on the cushion of the analytic couch. When I pointed that out to her, she replied that the (cushion's) "synthetic" material was harmful to her puppy.

At the same time, she kept complaining about the therapy. She said that coming to see me was a huge waste of time, and that she would have preferred to stay at home and have fun with her sister's friends. The truth was, instead, that she felt very vulnerable in that period, and she was often sad and lonely. On some occasions she started crying, telling me that it was because of the bright light in the room, which made her eyes water. She felt quite frustrated about her adolescent part, and at the same time she accused me of not providing her with a container, like a magic pair of boots that might allow her to run through life and to arrive first, without ever falling.

In the months that followed, Re abandoned the toy puppy and started to come to her sessions with a little purse and to wear brand new gym shoes with flaps. From her purse she would take out all kinds of things: coins, sweets, trinkets, and many other objects, which she got from a vending machine. Owning all those things and being able to show them to me made her feel wealthy and rich. This also allowed her to tell me that the vending machine was very generous because it gave her lots of precious things, whereas therapy took the best opportunities away from her. At the same time, she was literally fascinated with her shoes: she looked at them as she walked, tried changing her steps, took them off, stroked them, smelled them, bit them, and carefully observed their rubber soles. She seemed to be quite sure of herself with her shoes on. She felt brave enough to climb the stairs leading to the therapy room in big strides. One day I found her in the waiting room looking at the brand name of the shoes that two other children were wearing: triumphantly, she claimed that it was the same brand name as hers. This made her feel less lonely and broke the isolation and sense of alienation in which she felt imprisoned, and it also responded to her need to be seen just like any other boy or girl. However, she still complained about her being tired and empty, as if the things she filled herself with were not enough to make her feel alive and happy. And indeed they were not.

In the spring, on the occasion of a school trip with her class, she came to therapy looking quite distressed. She expressed her fear of getting lost during the journey, or of being left behind, all by herself, abandoned by her teachers. At that point she took out of her purse a brand new identity card. This allowed us to talk about her difficulties in feeling confident about her independence and of her mistrust towards her teachers, whom easily became unreliable people in her mind. In the following session we discussed the same topic again, but this time the identity card, which was still in her purse, was completely crumpled and hidden under a heap of dirty pieces of paper, which she had picked up from the street, making her document almost unusable. I made her notice how difficult it was for her not to hate that part of herself that felt dependent on other people, in this case her teachers, in order to feel safe, and how easily, instead, she relied on her more unhealthy part.

The therapist's dream

At the beginning of the final two months of therapy, Re began to regress, showing behaviours that were similar to those she presented at the beginning of her therapy. In the course of a session, in particular, she collapsed in her armchair, sticking her right thumb in her mouth without sucking it, while she brought one of her shoes to her face with her left hand, covering her mouth and nose. With her free fingers, she sometimes scratched the shoe. She did not look at me; her attention, all herself, apparently, was held together by this activity. I felt helpless and desperate, and after a while I was taken by an irresistible urge to sleep. I tried to react to this feeling, wanting to stand up, walk a little, and say something that might somehow break that silence; in the end, I fell asleep for a few seconds.

During that brief moment of sleep I had the following dream:

> There were three elephants near a palm grove in a desert oasis. They were walking in a single row, holding their tails with their trunks, as these animals sometimes do in a circus show. The last two elephants in the row started sinking, slowly but inexorably, into the quicksand. Only the third elephant, the first in the row, was already on terra firma, trying with all his might to rescue the other two.

This dream was important for a number of reasons:

1. From the clinical point of view, it helped me to modulate the constant oscillations inside me between hope and despair, and it gave me the opportunity to reach a more immediate and profound understanding of the pain and dangers faced by Re, which were linked to her definitive separation from therapy.
2. It made me understand that all the material about Re, which had been emotionally silent for a long time, had finally been worked through by my dream processes: in my internal world I had found a deep emotional link that seemed to put a definitive end to the experience of incommunicability of her solipsistic state and mine. This gave me the conviction that she had managed to stabilise an object, which was sufficiently attractive and strong to drag her out from the world of non-mentality, towards the world of meanings (the elephant that drags the other two out of the quicksand).
3. The dream gave me the opportunity to compare its compositional qualities to those of my analytic interpretative activity at the beginning of the therapy. I noticed that the images and the narrative of the dream, despite their simplicity—or even banality—were effective,

warm, and precise in their essential and complete expression of what was actually happening in that moment in the session. They had depth, concreteness, and realism even in their details (like the heaviness of the elephants, which reminded me of Re's movements when she seemed to be physically disabled), which made them deeply different from the images aroused in me by the patient's frantic activity in the past. Above all, they had an unsaturated quality, which constantly stimulated my imagination.

4. Finally, the dream made me understand that the image of the three elephants linked by their tails and trunks—the extended parts that Re had always cut off, leaving gaps and holes in their place—gave voice to a part of the child that said: "Let these links survive, because only they can oppose oblivion and mental death."

At this point I would like to remember what Meltzer (1984) wrote about in *Dream Life*, about the fundamental role of dream activity in supporting the ability to think; he stated that dream images perform two important functions: "binding" and "fixing" emotional experiences. In the first case, the emotional experience in the dream finds a way to be "named" through the encounter with an epistemological container. In the second case, always in the dream, the emotion that has become an image and a character is placed within the geography of the unconscious phantasy, thus favouring the distinction between the internal and the external world.

In child development, these functions are mainly performed by the mother. Through her alpha function and her reverie, she is actively engaged to find a name to the behaviours of her child and to fill with meaning their personal link. She initially assesses its meaning in the depth of her unconscious fantasy and experience, often through intuition, and then she returns it to him through verbal and non-verbal communications. Thus, she helps him approach the beauty of the world of emotions and thoughts, activating his imagination.

Similarly, in therapy, one can see that the "heart of the mystery" of the patient's mental life, her way of being and of experiencing life, starting from the analytic experience, is brought to light by the therapist not only with the creation of verbal or linguistic symbols, but also with the establishment of a scene. For these reasons, I believe that the therapist's ability to "dream" the infantile transference, as I did with the dream of the three elephants, belongs to the creative aspects of his mind and is very similar to the efforts of an artist who is busy with his work. The work of the therapist and that of the artist, therefore, come together in what D. Meltzer (1988) considers one of the fundamental functions of human creativity, i.e., to protect our passions, our imaginative thought, from the "cynical power of negative links" (Meltzer, 1988, p. 20) and from a "contractual adjustment to the world" (Meltzer, 1988, p. 140).

Commentary

This last year of therapy features, surprisingly, a positive evolution in Re's development. This happens in spite of the premature interruption. This positive development seems to be somehow linked to the resolution of child's geographical confusions in her unconscious fantasy and in the analytic infantile transference.

Initially, these confusions manifest themselves in the game of the perfumed puppy, when Re seems to personify a parental figure who looks after a part of herself represented by the puppy. The projective identification fantasy that supports this personification is much less intrusive and destructive than the initial identifications with the great big lady, the elephant, and the hairy man. After a few months of analytic work, the child is able to let go of her identification and starts to enter into another dimension, looking for safety through very primitive identifications with other children, boys and girls, by means of magical fantasies of belonging to one group or the other. The current adhesive identification with the group of peers (group mimicry) is different from the one she had expressed at the beginning of the second period of therapy, when she disguised herself with her "crazy hats". The envy, which accompanies the new fantasy of belonging, is less intense and leaves some room to more genuine feelings of pleasure and safety. In this sense, the school trip arrives at the right moment. She personally decides to take part in it, without knowing that, for a moment, her choice will take all her certainties away from her and will put her in touch with her paranoias. The experience of the school trip, outside any sort of protected environment with well-marked and concretely visible spaces, seems to anticipate the end of the analytic relationship which, however, will take place almost eight months later. On the level of her external reality, Re is asked to stand on her feet and to resort to her own internal resources while facing this new task and the anxieties connected to it. On the level of her analytic experience, this mental and emotional turbulence prompts her to a greater acknowledgement of her psychic reality.

Working on her identity card is important, because it helps Re to work through some of her paranoid anxieties towards her internal and external objects, and to discover that many of her manic aspects are linked to her attempt to strengthen herself, make a good impression and manage by herself, since the people on whom she might rely easily turn bad in her mind, either because they are "synthetic", or because they are damaged and hostile, due to her envious and jealous attacks. As the end of therapy concretely approaches, alongside the hope that a good internal link has grown stronger, there is also the fear that every positive experience may disappear in the vortex of confusion and despair and may be stripped of its emotional meaning.

Conclusion: the psychoanalytic method as an art form

I believe that the therapeutic experience with Re, a patient who certainly had a great artistic talent, together with the therapist's notes, can be seen as a continuous succession of sessions of life lessons in painting and sculpting (Williams, 2010a, pp. 122–131). In certain moments the therapist is the model for the patient, while on other occasions it is the patient herself who places herself at the centre of the therapist's interest and of his effort to comprehend her deep humanity, suggesting, with different poses, different interpretations of herself. This process includes movements, repetitions, variations, just like a dance, marking the passing of time. In this way, the roles of model and artist-observer become the expression of different mental states in the search for congruence. In the end, the shared form of the transference and counter-transference relationship in the mind of the two protagonists is beneficial to both, hopefully leading to an enrichment of their personal Selves and of their internal objects. The dream of the therapist brings forth a transformation in his personality, making him finally capable of helping the patient to start moving forward in her life again. The dream, like a work of art, reveals the integrating work of the therapist, who was able to transform the physical and emotional impact of the patient into a symbol, within a shared space. The clinical case of Re, as we also saw in the cases of T and S, confirms the fact that the main tool used by the children to talk about themselves is their own body, through movement, posture, and the way in which they position themselves in the physical space around them, passively or with passion, in a static or dynamic manner, relating to the objects they encounter. And it is with the body that they capture our attention, enchanting us with its shapes, gestures, movements, which seem to express a subjectivity that aims at manifesting and developing itself.

With their body, they draw something in the air, they create a sort of tension, a turbulence around them (Bion, 1970), something that is a pressing invitation to identification and knowledge, to the construction of a world of shared meanings. In other moment, however, as we have observed in the clinical material, the child is unable (or unwilling) to use her body to express something of herself: she prefers it to be like a passive instrument in the hands of somebody else; or she uses it to stage poses that are excited, pornographic, stereotyped, and noisy, which keep her distant form her real Self, preventing anyone present from thinking about her, making the activation of imagination very difficult, if not impossible.

PART III

IMPLICATIONS

CHAPTER NINE

The eyes and the mind (2): the exercise of knowing the self and the other

> "Now I would use as a model the diamond cutter's method of cutting a stone so that a ray of light entering the stone is reflected back by the same path in such a way that the light is augmented-the same 'free association' is reflected back by the same path, but with augmented 'brilliance'. So the patient is able to see his 'reflection', only more clearly than he can see his personality as expressed by himself alone (i.e. without an analyst)." (A note by W. R. Bion to D. Meltzer, quoted in 1986b, p. 121)

I

At this point in the research, after a long and arduous thinking on the written notes of the therapeutic experiences of Thomas, Suzanne, and Rebecca, we are faced with a considerable number of clinical phenomena that need to be organised within a unitary design: a few of them are well-known, others less familiar with uncertain meanings. Brought to light in the first instance by the dynamic forces of the analytic process, they have then been freed by what kept them hidden and that prevented us from understanding their nature. Now they lie on our workbench like precious minerals ready to tell us their story and the story of the ground that has preserved them for so long.

Beyond this metaphor the moment has come to bring together everything that we have learnt by the behaviours of the three patients within a complex and controlled setting, like the play room, and connect it to the actual, structural characteristics of their minds and to the ways in which they have presumably organised in the past, mainly in the perinatal period or early childhood, the flow of experiences in which they were immersed. In this way, the hope is to manage to reach a more truthful representation of their personalities, which may distance our judgement on their behaviours from the "*normality gap*" typical of psychiatric symptomatologic descriptions.

The clinical phenomena to which I refer belong to the manifestations of transference and are recognisable because they are metaphors of an emotional link. They must not therefore be confused *tout court* with the data collected in the three clinical histories, but should be linked exclusively to those "events" that have taken form within the analytical relationship and that have been recorded in my countertransference as products of the developing mind of the three children.

Without claiming to draw up a complete list, among the most relevant clinical phenomena that belong to them, I would mention: their bodily poses, between vitality, hyperactivity or dullness; their permeability to internal stimuli and painful external stimuli; the "no-entry" or "no-access" system of defences; the powerful even if limited force of their photographic memory together with the paradoxical transience of their ability to recall; the restricted and limited, at times really idiosyncratic interests that dominate their curiosity; the confusions between internal and external in the objects, between emergence and discontinuity in the background; the "special perspective" in the orientation towards the primary object of dependence; the overcrowding of characters, sounds or figures on the stage of the theatre of their mouths; the transient episodes of neck weakness (cataplexy) or sudden postural collapse due to general loss of the muscle tone; their excited and opaque states of isolation, and the peculiarity of their tears and snotty noses.

Among those that pertain to my experience in countertransference, I would mention: sudden attacks of irrepressible sleep and the experience of sliding involuntary into dreamless sleep ("the negative contagion"); the "confused" tone of my verbal communications, either too hard or inconsistent; the states of hyper-vigilance and mechanically recording details; and the wrong evaluation of the cognitive difficulties of the patients.

II

As a child psychoanalyst I am convinced that the type of participation that these patients—children and adolescents—enact within a therapeutic setting, precisely because it is built in the same way as the intimate relation of the new-born with the breast and maternal body, is bound to show what has been an "original disposition" in their primary object relations since the beginning of their lives.

The analytic session in this sense is the privileged place where the most unconscious levels of their mind, the most primitive mechanisms that underpin their mental processes, can be brought to light by the eyes of the therapist. Over the course of a psychoanalytic therapy I therefore expect to be able to discover, through my senses, "facts" of which I was unaware before, that are held in their movements, in their postures, in their bodies, in their attitudes towards the spaces, furnishing, and the atmosphere of the therapy room and towards my person.

These are facts that belong to that complex of experiences that, in the course of development, are the foundation of or ground the "*exercise of knowing the Self and the Other*" and the birth of psychic life.

In Chapter Three through the observation of the interactions between the "little rascal" and his mother in the intensive neonatal ward, we have had the opportunity to understand that "the exercise of knowing the Self and the Other" is present in the very early stages of infantile development, and that it takes the form of a *music-dance*, done by seemingly incessant comings and goings of notes and keys and rhythm, of different steps and moves back and forth We observed a small boy who participated in it with the movements of his body, his hands and his eyes, with the vitality and strength of his calls, his demands for care, while the mother, played the important functions of listening, reassuring, modulating, reinforcing and interpreting his behaviours and the external environment.

At the same time, in watching this music-dance between a very small boy who grabs his mother's finger and a young woman who sees into the future of her baby (as an adult he will be a "bad boy"), we are led to consider that the gaze of a child on his mother and vice versa is not simply guided by anxiety and need but also originally sustained by a particular "aesthetic" sensibility that has to do with the perception of beauty and emotional life.

Within the analytic encounter, psychoanalytic therapy therefore allows one to appreciate what even psychology and neuroscience have discovered in their research in the last fifty years on foetal and neonatal behaviour from the point of view of sociality and of the interest and motivations for the human connection, beginning from the maternal body, indisputably showing that in normal development the child is a precociously sociable subject.

Seen through this perspective, the clinical phenomena mentioned above do not leave any doubt that, over the course of a psychoanalysis with a child or an adolescent with pervasive developmental disorder, very different situations are encountered from the one that has just been described between the mother and her "little rascal".

The "facts" of which the therapist becomes aware in his counter-transference introduce him to the discovery of something uncommon and apparently incomprehensible, and that is to say that everything that normally creates proximity, contiguity and sympathy between two human beings, *even in the absence of a motivational conflict*, remains foreign to whatsoever interpersonal exchange, seemingly contrary to every experience of aesthetic reciprocity.

In accordance with that, I must say with conviction that the therapist who works with children or adolescents with pervasive developmental disorder should be well aware that he the will encounter numerous obstacles when carrying out its analytical functions. First of all he will discover how tiring it is, indeed sometimes impossible, to apply his intuition and imaginative capacity to the idiosyncratic behaviours and non-verbal communications of his patients. He will very soon give up the expectation of recording of the "natural" birth and growth of an infantile transference in the therapeutic process: rather, he will be confronted with unusual events that appear like moments of suspension of mental life and he will be in a position to see, even after years of work, the permanence in the personal link with his patients, of a disconnection between their personality and his own, and an irreconcilable difference between his own and their mode of participating in real life.

From the clinical material at our disposal, we can think that this state of affairs concerns the patients in the first place. Indeed, the three children, above all at the beginning of their therapy, appear to encounter serious obstacles in thinking through images, in expressing a subjective position through them; in remaining focused on their body and in attend the most common aspects of the everyday life, as if they did not know them; *"to turn a 'world of circumstances' into an opportunity for 'Soul-Making'"* (Keats, 1970 [1819]). Their mind appears disembodied and their body deaf and dumb, as if, as Meg Harris Williams says, "the rudder of attention is torn from the sub thalamic keel" of their mind (2010, p. 30), so that the oldest part of their emotional-sensorial experience does not couple the most evolved one.

At the same time we cannot overshadow the difficulties that I encountered as a therapist in understanding my countertransference. As we have seen in the preceding chapters, it has never been possible to use intuitively its contents to clarify the infantile transference of my patients however primitive or pathological. In a few stages of the therapeutic experience, above all the initial ones, my responses to the analytical situation, more than a psychological condition, appeared to be a condition connected to a bodily, sensorial, and perceptive bad functioning, or to a pathology of my brain (attacks of cataplexy).

It has not been at all easy to understand what universe of phenomena these experiences belonged to, either to the universe of "events or things" that we call "the brain" (on more than one occasion I have asked myself if by chance I were not physically "ill") or to the universe of processes that we call "mind" (a symbolic mind).

In more than one occasion I stressed the difficulty that I have encountered over long periods of time in carrying out whatever activity of thought on the psychological dynamics present in my relation with the three children, indicating as a specific factor that might have been responsible for it the poor quality of my attention and of the compositional aspects of my communications. With regard of it I remind you how my attention could in certain moments be turned off, inexorably extinguished like the flame of a lit candle in a place that is too humid and without oxygen, thus falling suddenly and irresistibly (by a sort of evil spell) into a mental state of dreamless sleep, a short mental blackness without images; or how, in other moments, my attention was substituted by a sort of automatic recording of reality, thus discovering, at the end of the session that I could recall, without any effort, in a vivid and precise way, all the details of what had happened (a sort of photographic or cinematographic knowledge of reality, whose memories-frames, in order to be brought forth, did not need the help of thoughts or emotions, something that we observed in Suzanne's behaviour before going to bed).

With the passing of time all my efforts to carry on my observations of the three children with empathy became impossible, and any attempt to identify with their behaviours was replaced by a powerful impulse to distance myself definitively from the living experience I was immersed. It happened that I felt a great impulse to find a secure shelter, either in the objective, scientific belief that nothing could be done to help them because their brains were definitively damaged (the opinion of Thomas's father) or in a faithful "vision" of psychoanalysis, that took the form of an interpretative monologue.

In this last circumstance, my way of communicating with children (temperature, speed, weight, consistence) could become so "broken down" that it would make it impossible to find the "necessary distance" between our personalities and an appropriate "language", verbal and non-verbal, that could sustain the birth and evolution of the transference.

III

All this brings back to mind the discussion that I left unfinished in the final part of Chapter Three, "The eyes and the mind", where I wondered why the attempt of Alessio, a high-functioning autistic adolescent, to share with me his ideas on the soul, and therefore on life and death, instead of making us feel closer, had had the opposite effect of making us feel more alone than we could ever have imagined, as if each of us had not found anything in the mental landscape of the other to hold on to (a sort of solipsistic drift).

My patient had been absolutely convinced of our immortality, on the basis of the religious theory of "reincarnation", and had made every effort to persuade me of the goodness of his idea. Over the course of the session he had transformed into an Australopithecus, and pretended to throw big stones at imaginary prey that was under the window of the therapy room. While he was playing the part of our common, distant and ancient hunter, he had looked into my eyes many times, in a pretty intense way, to monitor that I paid attention to him and was ready to understand what he wanted to tell me. Then, using his hands, in an awkward and erratic way, he had shown to me how the soul of the Australopithecus had entered into him, had concretely flown into his body. The meaning of message was clear but gestures and words did not manage to give substance to something that could be imagined as the house of this soul. Al's performance did not succeed to convey to my mind any idea of depth, neither in spatial nor spiritual term.

The charade that I had witnessed was at the same time comical and tragic, because instead of lighting up my attention, it had put me in the position of someone who finds himself in a colourless place tinged with a light that is too strong and uniform, where everything fades away, and whose eyes have nothing to hold on to. For this reason, I had closed my eyes in attempting to find within me an image of some importance to grab hold of that I could then share with him. Instead, without me being able to do anything, I had slipped slowly and inexorably into a dark gloom of dreamless sleep, as if I had been hit by an evil spell (the phenomenon of negative contagion).

Now we know, in the light of what we observed in the clinical material from Thomas, Suzanne, and Rebecca that the phenomenon of negative contagion, even though in different permutations, has sparked my conscience not as an exception but as the norm. We have moreover been able to verify that as soon as it has moved on from being a constant or started being less consistent within the analytic relationship, the capacities of the patients to develop and elaborate thoughts on themselves and others has increased. For these reasons, the clinical incident with Al, that I have just mentioned, becomes even more interesting if one compares it with what happened in the session of "the dream of the elephants", over the course of therapy with Rebecca, when the regressive behaviours and extreme isolation of the patient (who holds the thumb of her left hand on her throat while she rhythmically taps the palm of her left hand in front of her mouth like a wing), that before had produced so many moments of negative contagion, had finally found a representation in my internal world, in the way of a "dream thought".

If indeed we use the clinical phenomena of negative contagion and of the dream, as two vertices by which to view simultaneously the clinical material, it becomes evident that the focus of the session with Al lies in the fact that my patient's representation of the Australopithecus that throws stones has not been transformed into a dream thought in my mind. We can see from his performance that, beyond every consideration on the incompatibility of our personal points of view on the immortality of the soul, there is a sort of epiphany that does not find a way to reveal itself and to "become incarnate" in the therapeutic relationship. We have instead seen that the regressive behaviours of Rebecca, after having been muted and unthinkable for a long time, have finally sprang to life through the images of the dream of the elephants in the same way that the primitive behaviours of the premature baby, "the little rascal", had been immediately translated into a metaphorical language by its mother's love.

In the light of all this, the question on why the discussion on immortality of the soul had made both of us feel more alone than we could ever have imagined, leaves the room to the curiosity of understanding if there is something particular in the way in which Al represented the migration of the spirit of the Australopithecus within his body that could have contributed to switching off my imagination. The temptation is to attribute the phenomenon of negative contagion to the meagre quality of the material used by him in the construction or writing of the scene.

It is a hypothesis that does not however seem to find any evidence from the clinical situation observed in the session of the "dream of the three elephants". In fact, we can see here that the regressive behaviours and extreme isolation of Rebecca, (which in the past had made me fall into a sleep that was devoid of images and that now is transformed into a dream-like image in my mind), are identical on the phenomenological level. Instead, it seems to suggest the idea that the scarce quality of the materials and the links of actual representations are secondary to a developmental disaster that is re-enacted in the transference relationship.

We might think that the problem lies in the fact that the ways in which the patients use their own bodily experience to give form to themselves, which originally contained an emotional meaning, have then become, for some mysterious reason, so idiosyncratic, so elementary, so entrapped within the same script, to negatively affect our normal capacity to empathise with them. The initial search for the motives that lie behind the solipsistic drift, both of the patients and therapist alike, shifts its focus. It appears that our curiosity should be directed towards an understanding first of all of what might have caused that negative transformation in the course of the patients' development and then to what really takes play when, with the help of the therapist, the evil spell is partially lifted.

IV

At this point in the discussion we have brought together the evidence just for two truths, one clinical, the other theoretical.

The first one, based on the reliability of the psychoanalytic method, claims that the patients in session never stop trying "to find themselves", even when they seem completely lost in themselves and induce in our countertransference a death of our imaginative capacity. Moreover I think that the ways they express themselves, seen through a closer examination, even when they do not have the quality of a dream or an affective communication, may reveal "in transparency" something that belongs to their primitive bodily or relational experiences. By consequence, our job as therapists is, first of all, that of discerning those manifestations of a hidden life and of giving them a form that renders them visible and permanent (reanimating them), and, then, of locating them through our imagination and intuition in their original ground. In this specific case, one could think that my task with Al would be one of *finding the physical impressions of life in his soul,* because through his performance he shows the extent to which for him, the "soul" had been for a long time only a learned concept.

The second certainty, which is very important in my conceptual framework claims that the clinical phenomenon of *negative contagion* is ubiquitous in the therapeutic process with patients with pervasive developmental disorder. For this reason I think that one should attribute a syndromic meaning to it and that it should be studied as a specific factor in the disorder itself. Not only this: the fact that from a phenomenological point of view it configures a mental perspective or dimension that lies at the antipodes of an aesthetic experience allows us to consider it one of the factors of the alpha function working in reverse.

It is clear at this point how important it is to put oneself in the best position to recognise in the behaviours of our very ill patients those processes that belong to the first steps of the developing mind of normal infants and that reveal themselves in the exercise of knowledge of the Self and the Other. For this reason I decided in the course of my work experience to approach therapeutic sessions in two different ways, corresponding more or less to the two qualities of the attention I mentioned previously, one more active and the other more passive: respectively either as a sort of song and dance or a life-drawing class.

At the same time I trained myself to analyse the content of the material of the three clinical stories as if they belonged to a single biography, as if they were different moments, in progressive steps, of a single story, laid out in a spiral, by which little by little I could descend towards the bottom, then rise to the top, where the bottom had to do with the more primitive levels and the top with those more complex levels of symbolic development.

To have these instruments of navigation at one's disposal has served to protect my journey into these singular mental landscapes from the error of neatly dividing cerebral from mental events, running away too prematurely from the knowledge that the mind and brain are not only very complex in their respective phenomenological manifestations, but also profoundly connected to the other, in a very mysterious way (McGilchrist, 2009). This occurs above all when one finds oneself in the position, as in the analytical experience or in the natural observation of mother-baby interactions, of having the unique opportunity to glance at the most primitive levels of a child's development.

I think of the theme of the body in Thomas or the theme of language in Rebecca, which permits a journey from the bottom to the top or from the top to the bottom in order to understand the connection between bodily experience and symbolic development. I think of another journey that, following the theme of the geography of the mind (the "context"), connects our thoughts with Suzanne, half-way along the spiral, allowing us as we please to either rise to the top to the discovery of three-dimensionality with Rebecca, or to descend towards the bottom where we encounter an apparent absence of dimensionality with Thomas. We can in this way to have a better understanding of the reason why the discovery of symbolic forms in Rebecca develops itself through a complex process of push and pull. This hypothesis is based on the observation that what characterises our action at a distance in the link with an object that is different than us is made up of two movements: the first in the direction where we are pushed (the hands of the mother that bring the child to the breast) and the second in the direction towards which we are pulled, attracted, dragged forward, by aspects of reality that exercise a sort of magnetic force over us (the beauty of the face of the mother).

Only in this way, "seeing through in transparency" the clinical material, I have been able to discover, how much "timidity" was present in the bodily expressions of Thomas, thus transforming the brain-damaged boy in my mind into the little Boo-Boo bear; how much "greed" and "insatiability" were present in the movements of Suzanne, thus changing the image I had in my mind of her as the mentally retarded little girl into that of a spiteful little girl with golden locks of my imagination; or the degree to which a preoccupation with her own abilities and the beauty of her own attributes was present in the excited and wrongly displayed bodily behaviours in Rebecca, thus allowing the psychotic girl present in my mind to become the girl kissed by the Snow Queen.

* * *

At this point, after having discussed the conceptual and methodological tools that helped me to keep alive my interest towards my patients and to become engaged with them, the time has come to investigate "the forms of life" that I was able to find in their soul (their real Selves), the way in which they manifested themselves within the therapeutic process which I recognised in the traces they left behind in my countertransference.

For simplicity's sake, I will group them into three categories, of the body, the context, and the language, making references to the classical triad of impairments, in social interaction, imagination, and communication, as first described by Lorna Wing, that are shared by all people who suffer from pervasive developmental disorders and disorders in the autistic spectrum: the difficulty in having affective links with other people (paragraph v), the confusion between internal and external symbolic processes (paragraph vi), and the delay in development of verbal language (paragraph vii).

V

The "disembodied mind": the difficulty in building affective links with other people and objects

The claim that children and adolescents with pervasive developmental disorder have difficulty in building affective relations with other people, while finding apparently a confirmation in the description of some of the behaviours of T, S, and Re, seems to me a rather dangerous simplification of reality, for at least two reasons. On the one hand, because it favours a false equation of the "autistic" part of pervasive disorder with an "absence of the Other". On the other hand, because it does not take to far our attempts to understand what is really taking place in the course of the these children's development, when there are so many obstacles in their capacity to attend reality and to be empathetic in their communications, and how these impairments might have influenced their cognitive development and their social competence in the early phases of life.

The conception of otherness

If it is true that my patients, with their lack of interest towards me, managed on more than one occasion to make me think that what I was doing for them was useless and that it made little sense that I spent part of my time with them in session to the point of making me define the atmosphere that characterised our meetings for long periods of time as "deadly", it never happened that, confronted with "such indifference", I felt hate, reproach or refusal. On the contrary, I noticed that with the passage of time, as I learned to recognise and accept our "differences", without giving up searching for the right distance to observe their ways of being, my capacity to tolerate the weightiness of the situation improved.

That helped me to discover that the moments of isolation, when T, S, and Re ignored me or tried to deny my presence, in which they appeared completely absorbed in painful or, on the contrary, excited bodily sensations where they had an absent-minded and opaque, dull look, often alternated (perhaps even as a consequence of my therapeutic attitude) with other situations where "they opened their eyes" to reality, directed their senses and their attention towards me or things or events that took place within or outside the consulting room. I began to note that they were interested in different aspects of my body (my face and eyes, hair and glasses, my fingers), but also attracted by the spaces, by the atmosphere, the surfaces and by the light of the consulting room (I presume even the smells). In the end I came to the conclusion that T, S, and Re, despite how things might look, were in some way very much involved in the analytic process, and *a posteriori*, I can say that they have been involved since our first meetings.

That made it necessary to deepen the meaning of their difficulties in establishing a link with me, giving proper consideration to the fact that the three children showed some kind of participation in the experience that we were having together. In that way I was able to recognise that their behaviours, both of openness or closure alike, seemingly so different shared certain common characteristics. All of them indiscriminately suffered from "*restrictions*" and "*constrictions*". For example, they had to do with part objects, were based on limited and restricted interests that endlessly repeated themselves without great variation, not only impervious to every external stimulus but also that could disappear in a sudden and absolutely incomprehensible way, to give way to other interests that were just as idiosyncratic and repetitive.

All this has convinced me that the "autistic" dimension of their ways of being could not refer *tout court* to an "absence of the Other" or to a desire to cut off oneself from the Other, or be equated to a suspension of human mentality like the attacks of petit-mal, but was the consequence of a primary defect in their conception both of the Other and of the simple facts of everyday life, that prevented them from recognising and being recognised in the encounter with the Other and with Others, which they could not avoid in any way.

The vital link and the "vision" of reality

In order to understand the full meaning of these statements I propose that we should together follow what the three patients tell us of their primitive object relations, studying the manifestations of infantile transference.

First of all, we notice that those aspects that belong originally to "*looking at each other from a distance*" within the relationship of dependence of the child on its primary objects and that are revived within the analytical experience, are the first to suffer from "restrictions" and "constrictions". All my back and forth movements, both active and passive, with which I invite T, S, and Re to find a point of contact and of reciprocal recognition—holding them in my arms or putting them down on the ground, bringing them closer or distancing them physically from my body, catching their eye at a distance or estranging them with a rebuke, encouraging them to come closer or putting them down on the carpet—appear "disordered" and never take on a sufficiently stable, consistent, reliable, predictable or deep form such that can become the metaphor of an emotional link.

I think that this is due to the fact that the "feeling in memory" of the primary experience of breast-feeding (reactivated by the therapeutic setting) is not able to offer to this incessant flow of movements an anchoring to real life, a vital rhythm, and does not exercise on the patients an attractive and coagulant force that is both sufficient and safe. The compositional aspects of the infantile transference at this level are either saturated with persecutory and confusional anxieties and fantasies, or are dominated by feelings of urgency, impulsivity, of being out of control or of impotence so that they appear wrong in the rhythm, disharmonious, excessive in tone and speed, and unfit to carry out whatever form of emotional containment.

I remember on this point that all three patients have had a very difficult start to life that has made their first experiences of dependence on the mother's body and breast very problematic or impossible. T suffered from cerebral anoxia at birth, S was born prematurely and spent the first weeks of her life in an intensive care Unit, Re had instead a very depressed mother and a painful breastfeeding because of oral thrush.

The patients behave as if they did not have a conception of the breast-nipple as a good object. Their personalities lack a centre of gravity that makes them feel its pull of attraction both in the movements of coming closer and going away.

The main consequence of it is that *they cannot participate in a personal way in the relationship, as if it were a landscape*. The context within which the emotional link with the therapist should take form is continually perceived as a flat picture, which in its spatial elements lacks completely any geometric perspective.

On this point it is significant to observe how the patients' gaze, when it opens to the world, often goes further, beyond the gaze and the eyes of the therapist. It crosses the therapist's gaze to end up further, or stops beforehand, excluding it from the limited visual field that has been created, as if in their vision of reality were absent the conception of a nipple, the equivalent of a the "vanishing point" in painting or architecture, that may guide them in their movements back and forth the object in which they are interested.

Meltzer (1986c) maintains that the primary relationship between the baby and its mother on a part-object level is characterised by a double experience: *the first* one where the protagonists are the eye-nipple of the mother and the eye-mouth of the child; *the second one*, where the breast wraps up the new-born and the mother and the baby are both wrapped up in eye-to-eye contact.

> In the first case, the precocious discovery that the object can disappear from sight, and be unavailable immediately, activates in the new-born the desire to penetrate and control it with the eye and mouth. The collision with the will of the eye and nipple of the mother that prevents the baby from physically re-entering the

> maternal body and breast contributes to the tendency to split the nipple from the breast and to take on qualities associated eventually with the father and his penis that are characteristic of a very primitive and persecutory super-Ego […].

In the second case:

> […] the mutual envelopment of the aesthetic experience between mother and baby (and it probably must be mutual to be tolerable for a long period of time by either), with its passive, expectant and surrendering quality, brings the sense of mystery, of joyousness, but heavily freighted with the pain of the uncertainty of the aesthetic conflict for both. The hidden interior of the object, like the absent object, is a powerful stimulus to thought, perhaps the more anxious. While the anxieties engendered by the absence of the object tend to arouse violence in the service of domination and control of the object, the passion connected with the hidden interior of the aesthetic object promotes love-making, invites exploration. (Meltzer, 1986c, p. 183)

For the patients, in both experiences, the one of the "absent object" (in the sense of the breast that disappears and is not immediately available) and the one of the "mysterious present object" do not become a stimulus for thought and not activate the projective and introjection processes. In session, the primary and aesthetic experiences of feeding do not succeed in being part of the transference because they are too painful and are immediately evacuated, cancelled out in a violent and destructive way.

The flow of their perceptive and sensorial experiences in which they are immersed is therefore neither anchored in the concreteness and bodily feelings of the feeding experience at the breast nor is it sustained and vitalised by the aesthetic experience of reciprocity. This has a serious consequence on the image that with the eyes they manage to create of themselves, the Other, and the therapeutic link: it is a "disordered" image that lacks a unifying meaning, similar to a disembodied vision, "virtual" and not at all joyous, seen from a distance that is never correct and guided instead by special perspectives or points of view.

Even the experience of being looked at suffers from the same "limitations and restrictions". The children, through their postures and movements, do not succeed in finding an expression of the self, a human form, that is immediately accessible to those who observe them, as if the absence of integrated experience of the nipple of the surface of the body does not allow for the organisation of their subjectivity, and leaves a space only for adhesive identification (the spreading of oneself on the surface).

I often wonder whether the obsessive and repetitive features of my patients' tendencies should not be thought of as the expression of the lack of integration of the oral experience with the other sensorial experiences, above all the visual experience. I have observed, in fact, rare moments, when T, S, and Re seem capable of letting themselves be wrapped up by the beauty of the transference object, by the tone of its voice, by the light of its eyes, by the mystery of its mind. These situations, however, do not find an internal echo in their personality, they die in nothing as if they do not find a vital internal and personal relation capable of sustaining them.

"Watching from a distance" and "to experience the object"

These observations lead one to think that the "autistic" part is a form of "awareness" of reality that is born from a very particular way of seeing both oneself and others, that may be traced in a serious and primitive imbalance between the images of the maternal object, mainly the breast, seen by the baby through the senses, and the awareness of its presence and absence in the early phases of his or her development. For instance the way in which my patients, as it appears in the transference, look at the object from a distance is obtrusive of the possibility to "experience it". The movements of coming closer together/contact and estrangement/detachment that, with the help of the senses, normally lead the child to discover and look for the object as a different person from himself to be able to identify with, and help him to live, exist, and be known in a permanent way in a shared field of experience, takes on a different meaning in the experience of our patients. The attention which the child turns to the breast, face, and eyes of the mother that should allow him to participate in an active way in her personal landscape, stops itself at the external recognition of her beauty and her attributes, but never arrives at an understanding of her emotional qualities and her capacities to transform reality. It is as if the experience of dependence towards the breast in its bodily and aesthetic aspects, could never be integrated with the perception of it from a distance, above all the visual one. In this way the realisation of the combined objet gives way to "a misconception" (Money-Kyrle, 1968). The way in which patients looks at the object becomes so disembodied that the image that they create of it takes on the quality of a "belief" that contains nothing or very little of what they have experienced through their unique, individual and personal link with the mother as a part object: the primitive experience, vital and true of the dependence and separation from the breast becomes confused and substituted by a "vision". At the end of this journey as a support of their identifications and projections, there is the "vision of an object" and not the "presence of an object".

Countertransference reactions

All this becomes very significant if analysed in the light of a few, very peculiar, countertransference reactions which for variable lengths of time influenced my way of "looking" at the behaviours of T, S, and Re and which were also present in the parents themselves, or the teachers, when they watched the three children in their everyday life attempting to get to know them: situations in which the adults' observations, apparently punctual, precise, rich in detail and objective, in reality suffered from the same "restrictions and constrictions" that are present in the view of our little patients from a distance: they were too exact, too delineated, too scientific, quite disembodied and devoid of empathy and aesthetic sense.

I pointed out in the comments to the clinical case studies how I had observed that sometimes the experiences of my patients crossed my mind as sequences of single frames or moments of film, or parts of scripts recited in an often ineffectual way, that imprinted on my mind in an almost automatic way, producing sterile memories that did not activate thoughts or emotions. Paradoxically, even their tender and positive modalities of proximity had the effect of making me suddenly fall asleep, or better, fall into a mental state of "dreamless sleep", a sort of death of the imagination.

At the same time, I showed that in the moments when I succeeded in surviving their lethal impact and I found the enough strength to maintain an interest in these experiences and I began imparting to the memories I had of them an acceleration, or I tried to slow them down, in an attempt to locate and arrange them against a broad background (as when moving the probe of an ultrasound machine, one is trying to capture on screen the morphology of a foetus in the womb or, by changing the impact of the light, one tries to single out or imagine the details of a photograph that is out of focus because of a mistake in the exposure of light), *the images of what I had originally registered in my mind turned into forms of life* that reminded me of very simple motor and social behaviours, even though primitive and mysterious in their meaning, that belong to the normal development of a baby. *I could then see "within and beyond" the original script* something that recalled to me the images that run in front of the eyes of each of us when we observe the behaviours of a foetus in the womb in the final weeks of gestation, or of a baby during birth, or of a new-born stretched out on the floor of the house. On more than one occasion there was therefore the possibility of understanding the degree to which my way of functioning could reflect like in a mirror the way of being exhibited by T, S, and Re. Exposed as I was, for long periods of time, to the weariness of living through an experience poor or totally devoid of emotional significance, in my efforts to survive I ran the risk of letting the internal pathological objects of my patients become part of me, thus slipping into an attitude of *arrogant stupidity*, a particular form of omniscience that reduced the meaning of their behaviours to a simple concatenation of neurological events, or within a sort of *interpretative solipsism* in which I tenaciously held on to my psychoanalytic convictions and beliefs.

* * *

At this point in the discussion it could be interesting to pause for a moment and spend some time to re-read (to be reminded of some important features of) the clinical material in order to better understand how the three patients introjected some the therapeutic functions through me, when the more persecutory and confused aspects of infantile dependence on the breast were partly worked through in the transference.

We may see how the exchange of looks between the patients and me becomes a vital experience that allows to appreciate the reality of the Other and to reach at the same time a deeper awareness of oneself: the "necessary" distance is now present in the analytic relationship that permits a better understanding and expression of both one's own subjectivity and individuality (one's own emotions and transformative capacities of reality in which they participate).

One can find an example of it in in Thomas, who, after nearly a year of intensive therapy, takes on the challenge of willpower with me in an explicit and direct way; in Suzanne who during a separation, succeeds in drawing both my face and that of her school teachers in a recognisable way; and also in Rebecca who manages to create with plasticine a sculpture that clearly represents one of my three-dimensional images.

Thomas initially refused to look at me in the eyes; on the first occasion when that happened, almost by accident he burst into a very painful fit of tears, as if during the meeting between our two gazes something hard came out of my eyes and physically penetrated his forehead. Moreover, over the course of the therapy we observe that the child prefers to focus his gaze on luminous sources that are beyond and above my eyes: on the occasions when he fixes his eyes on me, he seems blind. His look is glazed. In contrast to that, on certain occasions he hides to let himself be sought by my gaze and then lets himself be enveloped for a few seconds by the light of my eyes. What is striking from the beginning in the case of Suzanne is that her great visual and tactile attention turned immediately towards my gaze where, however, she separated the high part that was felt to be good (the eyes) from the low part that was felt to be bad (mouth, voice). Rebecca initially appears instead to have a confused perception of my eyes that she feels at certain moments are like a protuberance and at other moments like a discontinuity (the topic of measles); furthermore, she keeps her experience of my gaze and my face that she considers good and enveloping completely separate from the low part of my body, genitals and bottom, that are considered dangerous and bad. Unlike the other two patients, she seems to be very interested in the "attributes" of my body and their functions, above all the sexual functions, to the point of not being able to recognise those vital functions that are linked to infantile dependence.

This summary of our longitudinal observation of the three clinical cases helps us to see more clearly, that when the therapeutic experience is perceived as "a good experience at the breast", "looking at a distance" returns to being part of that exercise of awareness that is fundamental for the birth of the mind, and it is no longer a "look that creates distances".

It is as if the perception of the object, at first inconsistent, fragmentary, distant, uncatchable, and dangerous, finally assumed the characteristics of a "gestalt", a stable "form", sufficiently complex, able to favour a minimum knowledge of the emotional and bodily processes and, consequently, the development of symbolic thought.

The clinical case of Re, as I have already said, is certainly the most useful to deepen these themes, in part because the baby was less damaged on a cognitive level with respect to T and S, but above all because there has never been any physical contact with her (as instead had been necessary with the other two patients, because of their motor disability), for which our relationship has developed only through the gaze and the voice. That helps to understand the extent to which it has been fundamental in this clinical situation to take care of the "compositional aspects" of my verbal communications and my mode of looking at her in order to favour the symbolic transformation of the experiences of dependence and separateness on the level of part objects.

VI

If it is true, as we have seen in the evolution of the three clinical cases, that the "autistic" dimension of pervasive developmental disorders (seen as a general poor awareness of one's own psychology and that of others) has to do with the fact that the actual experience of dependence on the breast, the nipple and the primary interest in the maternal body are in general replaced by "a virtual vision" of them, what can we say of the difficulties and the delayed mental development that our patients manifest on cognitive and social levels?

The clinical material of T, S, and Re seems to suggest that the deficit in empathetic communication, in the recognition of others as a source of identification, may have produced in their everyday life—above all in those contexts of human meaning like the body and the flow of sensations in which they were immersed—a failure to develop those processes that deal with the capacity to differentiate the external from the internal world (Meltzer), to have affective memory (Klein would call them "memories in feeling"), and to have a common sense view (Bion, 1963, p. 10) as well a common emotional view of an object (Bion, 1967, p. 119).

Previously I had affirmed that their behaviours, both those open to reality and those of a "no-access" kind, suffered from "constrictions and restrictions", showing how that state of things had at bottom a deficit of empathetic attention.

Now we can see that what takes the place which naturally belongs—from a developmental point of view—to empathetic attention, is another type of attention: it is an excess of an *awareness of reality*, for which, in everyday life, as it might be the case in very young babies or in foetal life, patients are acutely aware of facts, situations, attributes, and details of themselves and their objects that normally should be deposited in the unconscious and then remain active only on an intuitive level. For example, T and S are extremely sensitive to silence, to the minute variations of the atmosphere of the play room, while Re is acutely aware of details, of the attributes of the therapist and of herself. In addition, all three patients respond to what comes from outside or from inside their body or their mind, reacting disproportionally. On certain occasions, they behave as if they were devoid of a skin or protective filter, for which all their attention is grabbed and overwhelmed. In other circumstances, they behave as if their perceptive organs were flawed or absent, for which they appear deaf, blind or insensitive to physical pain.

The confusion between internal and external

W. R. Bion (1983) and Donald Meltzer (1986c), reflecting on the immaturity and the inadequate aspects of the structure of personality in borderline psychotic or schizophrenic patients, came to the conclusion that it is highly probable that normal children in the perinatal or postnatal development are "aware" of things which we adults have learnt not to pay attention to in our everyday life.

These experiences, instead of being unconscious, are objects of attention and the very young child would "feel that there is an intimate connection between his mental phenomena and those of others, animate or not" (Meltzer, 1986c, p. 177), and that at the same time that "he is not able to do 'anything' without having to notice and think about his actions" (ibid). In the very early phases of normal development, when there is a poor differentiation between external world and internal world, between imagination and action, between thoughts and facts, between Self and objects, the child's link with the flow of experiences that surrounds it, the exercise of awareness, would be overpowered by a sort of "bombardment" of mental phenomena and primitive perceptions, coming in a confused, changeable, fragmentary way from the internal and the external of their body, that does not permit a definition either of the self or objects.

"The wondering disability"

How can we imagine how a baby feels, sees, touches, and smells when this differentiation has not yet established? Where do processes of differentiation take place in corporeal experience? Is it taking place primary in the theatre of the mouth of which Meltzer speaks?

What is there in the child's most private and personal "reflections", that puts it in relation with the Other, that makes it feel close, in a context of differentiation? Is it the capacity of the child to transform "facts" into psychic "events"? Certainly. And on what is this capacity based, perhaps on the innate predisposition to appreciate the beauty of forms of life, to have feelings of wonder, amazement for them? It is therefore within its capacity to go "in depth", beyond the surface of things, through a kind of emotional turbulence that is aesthetic in its inception? When Alvarez (2012) wrote that "many so called learning-disabled patients can be found to have something more like an underlying 'wondering disability'" (Alvarez, 2012, p. 16), perhaps she grasped something essential in the differences between the development of a normal child with respect to a child with pervasive developmental disorder.

VII

What happens to a child that is only a few days or months old if it is denied the possibility to be amazed, to let itself be surprised, to become passionate in the encounter with the other, to feel the empathetic presence of another person next to itself, above all, the presence of the mother?

It is not easy to find an answer to this question. We know that the first days and months of life of my patients have been particularly difficult from every point of view, and on account of it, I am led to consider that the traumatic events, they have been through, may have created the conditions for that kind of "developmental disaster" of which I have just spoken.

The clinical material of T, S, and Re offers at the same time a few indications (perhaps more than one) of where we may find it. In this sense I am convinced that the answer we are looking for is inscribed in an indelible way in their body and language. We just need to look at them, as if we were examining the tree's growth rings, wanting to verify the presence of periods of drought and climate changes in the earth's history.

The "deaf and dumb" body

A close analysis of the modes in which the three children, through their postures, movements, actions, express their feelings and most primitive infantile impulses to grab and transform the external world, shows that their "bodies", unlike those of normal children, are "deaf and dumb".

There is no doubt that if we lay out our observations about it, disposing them along a longitudinal developmental spiral, we will notice from T to Re a progressive and autonomous sophistication in the way they use their body to express themselves. However, we cannot escape from noticing, that beyond their differences, their "bodies" never become instruments of a connection with the world or of an awareness that there is something more that lies beyond them.

We observe, indeed, that all the aspects linked to corporeal behaviour, either excited or depressive, lead both in the end to the same result: to their isolation. They seem to belong therefore to a same phenomenon, like two faces of the same coin. The exciting aspects are too deafening (T), too intrusive (S), or too fast (Re) to be able to be heard and to allow for communication, while the depressive ones are too low in tone, too slowed down, too weak to be heard.

Their "bodies" render "visible" an interweaving of depression and mania, that reminds me *of an automatic response* to a very primitive situation of danger, terror, and panic (Bion, 1982) from which one cannot escape if not through regression and flight into a foetal state, that in a regressive way seems to contain a catastrophic experience, otherwise impossible to take in. By looking closely at the bodily expression of all three patients, we discover that they represent two opposing reactions to a situation of intolerable panic. On the one hand, there are excitement and self-stimulatory behaviours, and on the other hand opaqueness, obstruction, immobility, and collapse. What is very interesting is their initial inability to express that terrible fear *with crying*.

The body of T is the prototype of the "deaf" and "dumb" body where the aspects of omnipotence and impotence collapse one within the other: it is a body that does not "speak", because in its flatness and immobility, the child seems silent and to have regressed to a foetal condition; it is a body that is "deaf" to every call, because the child is stunned and stunning at the same time as a consequence of his identification with a loud and deafening war machine.

Language and crying

As I was saying before, there is another place where one meets the developmental disaster linked to the "wondering" inability that does not allow the patients with pervasive developmental disorder to "see", to be "aware" that in reality there are two universes of phenomena, "facts" and "experiences", the physical entities and psychological ones. This place is the verbal language.

Keeping in mind that verbal language, compared to other mental functions, increases the capacity of the individual to dominate and transform reality and to hide or express the truth of oneself and others, the moment has arrived to discover the meaning of the linguistic behaviours in T, S, and Re, both from the expressive side and from the side that is receptive to listening, even taking into consideration the quality of "crying" as a very primitive but extremely important form of intersubjective communication.

Thomas (T)

If one casts an eye at the linguistic behaviour of T, considering only its executive aspects, the picture that emerges is somewhat painful; if instead we have the capacity to take an overview of it, some surprising and somehow unexpected facts are going to catch definitively our attention.

T is certainly the most deficient patient from the point of view of verbal production. On the expressive side: on a single occasion I heard him pronounce a word—"ava"—in an appropriate way and with clear intention, and I was able to observe joy in his eyes when I brought him a glass of water. Otherwise he only spoke in strings of two syllables repeated in a melodious way, for example, "pa ... pa, ma ... ma", within which he seemed to get lost. There is a single exception: in one of the initial sessions he articulated a whole phrase while I was putting his toy soldiers in a plastic bag. I do not recall his words because I was so taken by surprise by his speech that I had not time to record his words.

On a receptive level, he is very attentive to my words, not only to my tone of voice but also to their meaning, to the images they express. He perceives the tone of rebuke when I try to interrupt his stereotypes. His maternal grandmother recalls that he has always been fascinated by voices from the first months of life. He likes if you talk to him. He likes to hear verbal language. At the same time he is able to appreciate silence.

For T, in short, language has an "enveloping" function, it creates an indistinct relational situation, that makes one think of the experience of language that a baby can have in the womb or in its first few days of life: verbal language is not accepted nor is it appreciated in its functions of differentiation (the nipple).

The baby's crying comes at the beginning of the therapy session, a flat, indistinct, and repetitive "whining": it is exhausting, repulsive, annoying, and above all annihilating the possibility of shared emotional experience whatsoever. Subsequently, it will become a crying that communicates very painful persecutory and depressive anxieties, an expression above all of his feeling "lost" in the world, a feeling that stirs up a great tenderness in whoever is close by (Boo-Boo Bear).

Suzanne (S)

Her linguistic behaviour is complex, and complicated by bilingualism (English and Spanish). Within the family Spanish can be heard, while outside in the rehabilitation and special education centres that she is part of, people speak to her in English. She seems to have a good comprehension of both languages, even if she does not seem able to express herself in an adequate way using either idiom: her way of speaking is grammatically incorrect, a sort of word salad, or it is repetitive.

In any case, bilingualism has become intrinsic to some different aspects of her identity: she uses Spanish in a regressive, echolalic, repetitive and cold way in order to remain in the maternal world and estrange every experience of separation and of separateness from the mother; instead, she uses English as a symbol of weaning she links it to what is new, to changes, to what makes the difference between herself and the Other, to the metaphorical (fairy tale) and to the rules that help her to become independent.

The baby uses crying in the context of narcissistic processes of normal adhesive and projective identification: with crying she imposes her will, controls the object, makes her feel her own dissatisfaction and jealousy, and even succeeds in making her heard and understood by those who are nearby.

Rebecca (Re)

She has a language rich in vocabulary and correct in grammar, used very quickly, quick like lightning, incredible like whirlwind, fantastic and attractive like the syncopated rhythms of her play. It does not contain pauses but only sudden discontinuities. For this, when it is used to dominate and control interaction, it can become broken and fragmented. Words are absent, but so is the music, that part of vocabulary necessary to express feelings of loss of control, of falling into nothingness, into void, and of sadness and despair.

There is something that belongs to her most primitive and profound emotional experience that has no way to come out, to become visible, and to have a breakthrough in some expressive form of verbal and non-verbal language. It never finds its epiphany. No "poet" that might sing it. No "artist" who could represent it! It remains, instead, impossible to communicate and unimaginable, clotted in the regressive gestures of keeping her finger in the mouth or the hand on the eye, which are dense and idiosyncratic.

Re's tears never find a way to come out, her crying is frozen by anger, by resentment, by hate and cynicism that often transforms it into an "assassin's laugh", like the one that belongs to the Snow Queen.

VIII

The final observations on the body and verbal language confirm that all the aspects of personality of the three children, not only the link with the Other, suffer from restrictions and constrictions. We therefore need to apply, even to the operational activities, the point of view that we have used so far to understand the processes that underpin those clinical phenomena that have the meaning of violent and irreducible breaks in the dimension of the analytical relationship, which we would call affective.

In the previous chapters I suggested looking at these restrictions and constrictions—that should not be confused with inhibitions or neurotic limitations—in the same way as one looks at the changes in muscle tone and postural reflexes in childhood cerebral palsy.

I therefore expressed the idea that their effect on the development of the mind is comparable to that caused on the development of movements by changes to muscle tone and postural reflexes. I also pointed out that the restrictions and constrictions are the consequence of a disturbance of thought or a variant of thought, like the alterations of muscular tone and reflexes are "pathology" of the central nervous system. Continuing with the analogy, I considered the effort of a psychotherapist of "finding the physical forms of life in the soul of the patients", similar to that of the physiotherapist who, with the rehabilitating manoeuvres, tries to "paint a movement" (Quinton, 2002) in the cerebral structures of children, to increase the activation of normal sensorial-motor responses.

The study of infantile transference shows that the relation of dependence to the breast-nipple and the interest in the maternal body are substituted in our patients, above all in the initial phases of psychoanalysis, by moments of closing or opening to "reality" that apparently they look very similar on the phenomenological level to the behaviours of a new-born child or a child in the womb. The truth is, however, that they are fundamentally different from them, in the fact that in all circumstances they suffer from restrictions and constrictions that distort their profound meaning and become responsible for the clinical phenomena of negative contagion.

Moreover the exploration of the meaning of a few phenomena about which I have become aware in my countertransference, (like the "sudden falling" into a "dreamless sleep" and the "automatic recording" of events), have helped to discover that the patients are very different from us mainly in the ways in which they pay attention to reality or realise their identity.

Ways and *identity* here are similar but perhaps not identical to those which manifest themselves in the confused mental states of borderline-psychotic patients in Meltzer's cloistered worlds (1992) or in the delirious schizophrenic systems of pseudo-symbolic worlds, or worlds of concrete and symbolic bizarre objects of Bion (1962).

Indeed, using concepts of projective identification with part objects and the alpha function that works in reverse, it has been possible "to interpret autistic material in the same way that we interpret dreams" or better to transform it, to insert it into a narrative context. The experiences with T, S, and Re are there to demonstrate how difficult it still is in therapeutic practice to fill in the distance between clarity that concepts introduce in the understanding of clinical material and the possibility of "dreaming" the mental states of these patients in a transformative sense, as happened with the dream of the three elephants in the clinical experience with Re or with the story of little Goldilocks with S.

Perhaps we still know too little of the ways in which perception of mental qualities work in the links between people, and of the relationship between attention, movement and language in the development of the mind.

While I write this, I think to what could have led to these positive results: I think that artistic talent and intelligence has played an important role in the case of Re; the great determination to look for "food to eat" in S to a breaking point of violent moments of wilfulness.

I think above all that someone before me, the teachers in the cases of T and Re, and the mother in the case of S, must have fought with all their strength, without ever entirely giving up, for many years and in different contexts, against the inclination of the three children to break every emotional contact with people and reality, and they achieved this through continual confrontation, and by uniting and guiding the various aspects of the infantile Selves of the children towards a goal, preserving their vitality and force.

I have always felt that the various aspects of the infantile Self of the two children functioned, even if in an undifferentiated way, with the compactness and force of a *rugby scrum*, when players prepare to hook the ball to carry it towards their goal by fighting against the pack of the opposing team.

At this point I remember as if it were yesterday the moment when finally, through drawing, the various aspects of Re's infantile Self presented their credentials on the stage of the theatre of therapy: they had a lively charge, bursting through, similar to that which I can imagine belongs to the will of a rugby player.

IX

"Exit"

I would like to finish this chapter by talking once again about the main characteristics of the three children that, as we have hypothesised, are pervasive in every aspect of their personality, applying what we know about them to the most objectified aspect of development: the cognitive dimension.

As you have had the chance to observe in the clinical material, the three children, before beginning psychotherapy, had been subjected to a battery of tests and instrumental neurological exams that showed the intellectual level, the condition of the brain and the functioning of the senses. I had at my disposal a very reliable and complete assessment of their dysfunctions that would help to be objective in evaluating their working and social behaviours.

In the reality of the experiences in therapy, I was confronted with the discovery that children can be cognitively retarded and socially unsuitable in two ways: firstly, when they were lost or prisoners of their ways of being and ways of identifying themselves as "disembodied" (the theme of restrictions and constrictions returns), the second when they behave as if they were younger children than their actual ages.

On the cognitive level the first mode generates something very similar to that which I described on the emotional level: everything that would normally unite two people on an intellectual level made us feel distant and alone as never before. When instead they behave as if they were younger than their actual ages, I was able to feel all their weariness and their suffering in needing to confront the adventure of life while unarmed, poorly equipped, and "unaware".

In the light of these observations, I believe that it is appropriate to look at a few situations that are very much representative of these two modes of being "cognitively retarded".

Let us focus on S leafing through the yellow pages when she was sat at the seat of the "great big lady" with the ways she plays with her hands at the children's table; T's certain movements (bottom shuffling and lying prostrate) with the sense of disorientation that he feels at the moment when he gets to his feet and decides to walk by himself; the explosive narrative of Re's three Jewish stories told with her wavering when she points me to the news story of the little child who succeeds in escaping from the cot that is on fire We can also contrast the ease with which, on leaving the play room, S walks on her mother's steps, with a loss of memory of the room that after the holidays became for her a completely unfamiliar place; the excitement and auto-erotic exaltation of Re with her "little girl" ways of creating an adolescent identity.

Conclusion

At the end of this chapter that has cost me a great deal of energy, I could not say that if what I wrote had a certain value from a scientific point of view, and if it could effectively contribute to improve the current or future understanding of the ways of being of children and adolescents who suffer from pervasive developmental disorder. As far as I am concerned, I have only the certainty that today I still feel very ignorant on the subject. I hope however that I have been able to convey to the reader my commitment in working on the clinical material with my rugby scrum: it has been a hard battle on the field.

CHAPTER TEN

In the clearing of being: the difficult discovery of shared meanings in the process of weaning from therapy in a patient suffering from pervasive developmental disorder

Foreword

In this final chapter of the book I would like to consider the concepts of "treatment" and "cure" in psychotherapeutic and psychoanalytic work with children and adolescents suffering from pervasive developmental disorders. I shall do this by focusing my attention mainly on those aspects of their personality, stemming from their mental functioning, when they recover from being autistic or psychotic.

The importance of this study is linked to the fact that even after years of therapy, we must acknowledge that there is something irreducibly peculiar about their mode of being. We find above all in their character a mixture of immaturity and obsessional traits (Hoxter, 1975), which is difficult to interpret on a developmental basis. As such, we are eager to learn how much of it represents an overcoming of the initial condition or simply a sophisticated transformation.

As a basis for my discussion, I have selected the written notes of five sessions of the last year of Al's therapy, the adolescent patient suffering from Asperger's, whom we have already met in Chapter Three, when I talked about the countertransference phenomenon of the "negative contagion", which occurred during our discussion of the immortality of the soul.

I am deeply convinced that stopping to reflect on what happens during the concluding sessions of a psychoanalysis, (when, as we know, a special light is projected on the therapeutic relationship from the child's infantile transference activated by the ending), is like taking a rest at sunset in a glade, through which one has passed many times before, the difference being that there is now a different light that it broadens and exalts one's vision and allows one to see something new, more beautiful and mysterious, in everything one presumed of knowing very well.

My hope is, therefore, that pausing in thought in the clearing of the five sessions may enrich not only our understanding of the actual salient characteristics of the personality of my patient, who is just finishing his therapy, but also help us to discover new meanings of the main symptoms which were present at the beginning of his illness, such as isolation and the delay in the symbolic development.

Introductory notes

Al finished his therapy at the age of fifteen-and-a-half, almost sixteen. He was sent to me from the family paediatrician at the age of four-and-a-half, after having been diagnosed with autism. Since then he has undergone psychoanalytical therapy with me, with no breaks at all, for around ten years. During his time at nursery school he came five times per week. Following this, when he started junior school he came only three times per week, which lessened to twice a week during his time at secondary school. After the final summer holiday, in his tenth year of therapy, his family suggested that we start thinking about finishing the sessions; it was then decided that we should end it by the following summer. At that point Al started coming only once a week.

The five sessions, which I will discuss, in detail, are from the final period of Al's therapy. The first session took place straight after he had been told the end date of his therapy. His remaining sessions were to continue weekly following this. His second and third sessions took place close together, during the final six months of his therapy, and the fourth and fifth are, respectively, the penultimate and final sessions he had with me.

The first two years of therapy: the analytic period

Before presenting and discussing the clinical material, I would like to suggest to first read some notes from the very earliest period of therapy with Al, from age four-and-a-half until he started school at the age of six years and seven months. I believe that these notes may well be useful to get an idea of the evolution of his personality across the years; to compare, in a constructive way, the way I imagined him at the beginning of his treatment with what emerges from the clinical observations in his last year of therapy. Moreover I hope at the end to be able, from the study of the transference in his adolescence, in the "clearing" of the sessions, which will later be described, to show a fresh understanding of the meaning of his past behaviours.

These are my notes from the earliest period of analysis:

> Al is coming to see me for his session every day, with the exception of Saturdays and Sundays. The hope is that analytical therapy may rekindle his interest in the lives and minds of other people, making it more consistent; all the expectations are that it may help him at least partly to catch up on the delay that he has accumulated in his development, compared with that of his schoolmates.
>
> He is an isolated child. He spends most of his time lost in a world of his own either absorbed in repetitive, imitative, and idiosyncratic activities, or else falling victim of violent tantrums, full of angry demands or cries for help. As his mother would say, he seems to live in a bubble.

Here is a reconstruction of some typical movements of Al during the sessions of this period of therapy:

> Al is always alone when he comes up the stairs leading to the office. He follows his mother from behind, never holding her hand and never speaking a single word to her. He goes straight to the play-room without saying goodbye to her. His mother settles down in the waiting room, where she spends all her time embroidering a doily.
>
> The child is always holding something. In his right hand he keeps a white paper tissue, which he uses to blow his nose or to wipe food from his mouth. In the other hand he usually holds something to eat, such as a piece of chocolate or an ice cream.
>
> He never makes eye contact with me, but he sees me; he does not reply when I greet him, but he hears me; he follows the direction of my gestures, but he does not take my hand. His steps are sure when walking towards the therapy room. He betrays no hostility, rage or even anguish when he ignores me.
>
> He seems to act as though he wanted to remove any diversity, or as if he did not have an internal landscape in which he can position me or find

a living character in his internal world that he may associate with me. As such, there is no possibility of recreating me through his imagination and therefore to search for me as a transference object.

He quickly makes use of the other spaces of my office, such as the waiting room and the bathroom, where he often goes to urinate. When for any reason he leaves the room, he has no difficulty finding his way back.

He is not frightened when opening the toy-box. He rummages through the toys or sorts through them, as if he already knew them or as if he were looking for something in particular. He doesn't ask me anything and he doesn't show me anything. He doesn't complain; he simply ignores me.

In the main parts of the sessions he spends time repeating the same games or the same movements over and over.

Occasionally he spends a lot of time playing alternately with two small toy cars, a yellow one and a red lorry, which he found in the box, rolling them forwards and backwards as if he were trying to park them.

At other times he walks up and down the room for entire half-hours, his head bowed, always making the same route between the window and the door. He gives the impression of being lost in deep thought. Otherwise he stands on a chair and begins to incessantly clean the windowpanes, never speaking and never showing the least interest in my words.

At other times he curls up on the ground, near to the couch, and spends his time stroking the bars on the side and ridges of the springs, squinting at them from close range, treating them almost as an object he was observing under the microscope. He is helped in this activity by two soft toys, a little bear and a puppy, which he also forces to explore the couch.

Following this, he starts to spin around, making dance-like actions with his body and head, very similar to the movements of the silkworm when it weaves its cocoon. He spins around for minutes on end, without ever stopping, leaving me astounded that he never loses his balance.

There are also times when he spends all of his time smoothing, in every direction, the creases of the couch coverlet, or picking out very carefully its loose threads.

Lastly, he tries to act out something, which there and then I cannot seem to understand. It is some sort of complex scene or story, which only he knows, and he acts it out endlessly, without ever stopping to explain the meaning to me. It is only after a few months that I discover directly from his parents that there is one particular scene which he loves: it is connected to the episode in the film *Back to the Future*, in which the character Emmett Brown (aka "Doc"), at a very precise time indicated by the bell-tower clock, manages to reverse the direction of time, capturing the energy of a lightning strike.

When he is told that the hour is about to come to an end, he throws everything haphazardly back into the toy-box, leaving just a small space in a corner, where he leaves his dirty and crumpled paper tissue, which he pretends to find during the next session. He leaves with no fuss at all. He ignores his mother: when he finally re-joins her in the waiting room, he immediately absorbs himself in acrobatics on the arms of the sofas, or else he starts to play silently, brushing against the radiator. He apparently feels no anguish, and shows no other emotion. He is elsewhere. As his mother says: he is in his bubble.

I wonder what his "acting" means. Al, certainly, wants to erase any awareness that he is in a place other than his home, and he feels a powerful need to fill any space with a character that he already knows very well. At the same time, I see him both as an actor and a prisoner of the characters and the "scenes" that he chooses to act out.

Why doesn't he share the significance of his "scenes" with me, becoming a metaphor of our link to one another? How are they all solipsistic in nature, the embodiment of a helpless automatism?

I try to understand what the relation could be between, say, the original scene of the film *Back to the Future* and the one which Al is now entertaining in his mind. Why doesn't the "scene" that the child acts out on the stage of his therapy room seem to me to be an imaginative act of his mind? And why doesn't the child himself appear to me like one who is thinking through the "scene" he is acting? Which characteristics has the "scene" acquired in his mind, that it is capable of endlessly imprisoning him?

Whilst thinking about all of this, I start to note after a few months of therapy that his "autistic behaviour" or "obsessive flattening of every new experience" starts to enter into the "analytic" discourse.

The child seems to react to my frames of mind, and above all to the quality of my attention and interest in him. His "being far from me" automatically manifests itself when I do not manage to "survive" the lethal repetition of his behaviour, and to maintain an interest in him and in the things that he is doing.

This contradicts my beliefs that a child suffering from autism is unable to experience emotions or to some extent to tune into the frames of mind of those closest to him. At the same time, I begin to feel with some conviction that Al doesn't expect that he is or can be a "lovely child" and also that he does not sufficiently trust that he is protected by me or that he is safe in my hands. He does not seem to think that his presence can excite me, that his therapist would come to life at the sight of his smile, really develop an interest in a game or a joke that he is playing. It seems as though he is only expecting to be asked for the umpteenth time to "be perfect", to be on top of it, to be sure of himself, to be obedient.

I arrive at the conclusion that "to be a lovely child" has no place in his interior experience in the relationship he has with his internal objects. He must simply be a "good boy", "well-behaved", who must not "drop the ball". This is most noticeable during the times when Al sits on my lap, or when I hold him in my arms to take him around the room in an attempt, perhaps a clumsy one, to create a closeness with him, a shared common interest.

In these situations, he usually avoids meeting my eyes and looking at me: in those rare occasions when he meets my eyes, he fixes me for several moments with an intense, homicidal stare. I don't then understand if my eyes or, better, my pupils represent for him a black, dangerous tunnel, or else an emergency, which, like a cork, blocks any access to what is beyond. As for me, I feel an intense physical pain if I try to meet his eyes, as if an opposing force were stopping me from bringing them into focus.

At the same time the child, when he manages to stay on my lap for several minutes, experiences a different sort of intimacy with me than the contact with his eyes would suggest, but it is a very tender "maternal" attention. He begins to carefully tidy me up, rearranging my collar and smoothing out the creases in my jumper. This behaviour immediately stirs a paradoxical response in me: instead of feeling closer to him, I am gripped by a sudden sleepiness, which I find difficult to resist (I have a sort of narcoleptic attack which I called "negative contagion").

There is something odd in his movements, or in the "maternal" identification, which sucks out the life from my body and soul (which reminds me the emptied apple in Rebecca's clinical material), like the magic of an enchantment, which quietens every turbulence (like the voices of Ulysses' Sirens). *Perhaps it is the same thing, which transforms the "scene" of the film into a first draft devoid of any emotional resonance.*

There is, finally, another group of phenomena, which seem to be linked to a sudden decline in his defences, usually from exhaustion or from a fear of punishment. I often witness a sudden and catastrophic failure in his muscle tone. At these times Al takes on postures and regressive movements, typical of a much younger child. His movements are uncoordinated, where the muscle tone becomes as floppy as that of a ragdoll. Otherwise he strokes himself or lies face down on the floor or on the couch, without really being able to move forward or backward. As if he were masturbating.

Only once did I approach him while he was strenuously writhing around on the floor, to check that he was not having an epileptic fit (not that he actually suffers from them). This provoked terror in him just like our previous eye contact had done.

At other times Al pretends to be helpless, or starts walking on only one leg, imitating a person with limited mobility. He also lies on the ground, immobile, pretending to be dead.

Does he want to show me how "witty" he can be when he is acting out these little scenes, or does he perhaps want to show me something that really frightens him? In these situations, I often think about the painful scans that he underwent during his first two months of life, caused by an anal fistula, which thankfully closed up on its own without the need for surgical interventions.

Seven years later … the last year of therapy

I will begin with the clinical material compiled during the sessions, which followed my revelation to Al that he would soon finish his therapy, and the transition to only one session per week. I recall that he, at this point in his therapy, was close to his fifteenth birthday and is in his second year of a scientific lyceum (high school), where he follows a personalised teaching programme.

Alessio (fourteen years and eleven months)

He arrives on time, loaded with stuff.

Rolled up under his arm, glued to his body so that they cannot fall to the ground, are a fleece and a mackintosh. In his right hand he holds the wooden stick of an old ice cream that he has already finished, a crumpled tissue with which he sometimes tries to wipe his mouth and nose. In his left hand he is hiding an ice cream, still in its colourful wrapper. He stops at the entrance and makes eye contact with me; his gaze is a little strange, and seems to me to be directed inside himself, rather than at me. His eyes are opaque, as if they were veiled. Every so often he pulls a face, twitching and smirking. With the hand with which he is holding the wooden stick, he pretends to measure his nose up to mine. He tells me that our noses are level with one another, and that he has grown this week. He notices, however, that the stick is not exactly horizontal. He corrects it and verifies that my nose is, once again, at a higher position than his own. Then he rushes to my side, and stands against me shoulder to shoulder. Again, for a moment our shoulders seem to be level. Then as soon as I have reassumed a more proper posture, straightening my back to head towards the therapy room, he slowly but surely sees the contrast and discovers that our statures are indeed different and not, once again, in his favour. I am certain that he wants to immediately obliterate the awareness of this difference. He lengthens his neck and stands on tiptoes, but the many objects he holds in his hands prevent him from doing so. He thus launches himself towards the therapy room, inspecting himself in the windowpanes (it is already dark), which are right in front of him. He seems disappointed to have discovered that he really is shorter than I am. After having looked at himself for several seconds, he turns and says to me: "You see? I've grown because I've drunk so much milk", pointing out that the ice cream which he holds in his hand is milk-flavoured. He seems like a comedian. At this point, I jokingly say to him: "Do you think it's time to actually greet one another?" I say hello to him. He laughs and replies with a "Hi". He throws what he no longer needs in the bin. He puts his fleece and mackintosh on the table. Then he quickly leaves the table to go to the toilet. He comes back almost straight away with a clean sheet of kitchen towel. He begins to unwrap the ice cream. He devours it in large mouthfuls, and keeps looking at himself in the windowpanes. He repeats to me, with his mouth full, that he has grown this week, all the while trying to find some sort of proof reflected in the glass. He comes closer to inform me that my shoes have a sort of wedge heel, and compares them to the soles of his own shoes, saying that his are only half a centimetre tall. He lets himself slip onto the couch for a moment. He is so tall that he has trouble stretching out and finding a comfortable position. I point out how difficult it is for him to lie on the children's couch, since he has grown so much over the last few months. He says in a low voice: "You think I'm a shrimp!" I reply to him that it seems difficult to imagine how I could call him a "shrimp", since he is over five and a half feet tall, which is taller than most people I know. As if I hadn't spoken, he gives me the usual spiel of how before the summer he was five and a half feet tall, then after a month he was five feet and seven inches tall, etc. He quickly gets to how he is now over five feet nine (taller than I am) because five months have gone by. I have to resist the urge to flippantly tell him: "That's maths for you!" At this point I tell him that the measuring stick with which I checked his height recently does not correspond to his calculations. I remind him that according to the measuring stick, he is still shorter than I am. I add that I would be willing to measure him in a few weeks and that it wouldn't bother me if in the meantime he managed to grow so much that he ended up taller than me. I remind him, quite peremptorily, that the case of his height is closed, commenting that he can't get away from what the measuring stick says.

At this point Al jerks up from the couch and goes and puts the wrapper of his ice cream in the bin. Then, dissatisfied, he takes out of his jacket pocket more packaging of an old ice cream he had eaten the week before. He also throws this in the bin, with the air of someone who is acting respectably. I notice his actions are full of the same resolve as my voice had been, a moment before, when I shut down his talk of our respective heights.

He does not go back to the couch. He sits at the table, where he starts drawing a rainbow with his colouring pencils. He stops when he reaches the sixth arc. He looks at his sheet and then at me, starting to repeat "indigo, indigo", disproportionately prolonging the first syllable of the word: "Innnnn … digo". With the air of someone who has some precious information, he explains to me that indigo is a mixture of blue and violet (in the prior sessions he had carried out several experiments with these two colours to make indigo). I note that today he is only drawing with his right hand and he does not seem to need to redo the rainbow with his left hand, as he had done with all of his drawings in previous sessions. Today he does not seem to need to show me how "special" he is, one of the "few people" who are ambidextrous, like Leonardo da Vinci. He traces the violet, drawing each of the colours of the rainbow again and again, mispronouncing "orange" and saying the word "indigo" in his strange way again. He laughs and looks at me when he says "orange" wrongly. He seems satisfied, on one hand, at his ability to play around with words, distorting them and giving them a "countrified" accent, and, on the other hand, he is pleased at knowing less common words. I stop him by telling him that his constant repetition of the same joke, intended to make him seem interesting, gets boring after a while (I phrase this more sensitively). He is amused and repeats the word "boring". I remind him that in the previous session we had spoken of the rainbow as a natural phenomenon which signals the progression of the bad weather to the good weather, of the storm to the calm, the return of the sun after the rain. I ask him if he ever noticed anything similar to the arrival of the rainbow in himself. "How many times", I ask him, "have you been nervous, confused, angry at the start of the sessions, and left as calm as the sky is after storm … perhaps you find something here which makes the sun come back in you, and which makes your bad moods go away!" Al finishes drawing the rainbow, seemingly uninterested in what I said to him. He shows me the finished drawing and straight after, seems to connect with the fact that I mentioned the bad weather, and starts to ask me if I agree that it rains often in November. Moreover, he wants to know whether it rained more last November than it had rained this November. I repeat that I am not a weatherman and that he is far more of an expert in these things than I am. Undismayed, he continues to shower me with these questions, until I make it clear that I will no longer listen. I pretend to cover my ears. He looks at me and laughs, thinking for a moment that I am only joking, and then when he realises that I actually do not want to listen, he approaches to take my hands away from my ears. He is now sure again that I can hear me, and teases me by asking me the same questions again. I tell him that he is a real bore. He goes to sit down and in a pleasant tone begins to repeat, with lots of embellishments, things like "I don't give a toss about Dr B". I tell him that I am convinced that the fact he feels he can say such mean things to me, joke around with me, and talk in a "countrified" way with me just like the actor Gigi Proietti does in his adverts for Kimbo coffee, should make him feel OK, and put a smile back on his face, making him feel calm again. He sits at the table again. Whilst he is putting the finishing touches to the arcs of his rainbow, he starts to ask me whether rainbows can also be seen in winter. I reply, telling him that the observation behind his question about whether rainbows can be more easily seen after summer storms than after winter rain seems very interesting to me. I ask him if he would be able to give me an explanation of this phenomenon. He immediately replies: "Pass". I say that even I wouldn't be able to provide an explanation for the natural phenomenon, which he observed, and I attract attention to the fact that he has been capable of passing the question to me when he realised that he didn't know the answer. I remind him that when he was little he never accepted the fact that he didn't know or understand something, and would be so embarrassed about his ignorance that he would pretend to know everything and never ask for explanations. Then, changing the subject, I ask whether life for him is a quiz. He replies, convinced: "Yes, life is a quiz". I suggest to him, then, that not knowing, not understanding, or a wrong answer, carries with it the same risk in his life as missing out on a prize at a game.

This is just like what happens to the competitors of the famous game on TV that he watches so often: getting a wrong answer means being eliminated from the game, losing any chance of winning the prize or of going back to play again. I remind him that the "elimination" had been the term he had used when he referred to our cutting out the Friday session, when it was decided that we would meet just once a week. I tell him that I am trying to understand if, for him, the end of our therapy sessions was linked to a kind of permanent elimination from winning a prize at a game. At this point, Al begins to violently and insistently blow his nose. He shows major signs of impatience at this unexpected cold and does all he can to get rid of it. I make him take note of his impatience, maybe through anxiety at what is happening to him, which resembles some sort of unexpected climatic change. He makes no reply. He is too busy noisily blowing into the tissue or cleaning inside his nostrils, staying seated on the chair. Then he gets up and goes to lie face-down on the couch. He seems to have found a way of making up for the internal pressure in his ears. In pulling himself upright, he notices by chance the reflection of the window (through which the light from the streetlamps is pouring) on the wall of the room. He is visibly curious about it, stays sitting and brings his fingertips closer to the bright part of the glass, as if he wanted to probe the material or else feel how hot it was. Then he starts to move his fingers and to look at the shadows, which are forming on the walls. In the meantime his cold has vanished. He makes shadow puppets for a few seconds, and then he stretches out on the bed, in a supine position, without ever looking away from his fingers, which carry on moving like tentacles. He continues for a while to look alternatively at his fingers moving and at the light, lit in the middle of the room's ceiling. Then he finally stops to look gaze closely at his fingers for a long time: his smile is tense as if he were trying to arrange his fingers in a very precise way, but can't manage it. I am reminded of him playing shadow puppets when he was little, when he tried to re-enact the scene of a cartoon in which there was a witch riding a broomstick, which flew in the air, before being forced off the broom and, in the end, thrown head over heels to the ground. Or else his movements when, supine on the couch with his face turned towards the ceiling light, he would play shadow puppets for a long time, moving them like tentacles, close to his eyes. I speak to him about my memory of his past behaviour, in the hope that I will glean a comment, which will help me to understand it. Al, however, seems to be more interested in other things, in other worries, which he favours over me. At this point the session is over. I move closer to tell him so. He gives me a look of agreement. Despite this, he does not rise. Rather, he stays stretched out on the couch and starts to play with his fingers in front of his eyes, recreating the scene from *La Vita è Bella* (Benigni's Oscar-winning film) in which Ferruccio, the poet, talks to himself, repeating the prophetic, hypnotic command: "I'm sleeping, I'm sleeping", to show his friend Oreste that he is already in a deep sleep and so he can't get up from the bed to turn off the light. Just like this, Al pretends two or three times to fall asleep and to wake himself up, using just the magic of his hands. Then, prompted by me, he gets up. Without saying goodbye, he heads off towards the bathroom as usual. Arriving at the door of the therapy room, he turns back and uses the palm of his hand to stroke firstly the seat he was sat on, and then the part of the couch where had been stretched out for so long, as if he wanted to feel the heat that his body had left on the objects.

Commentary

I believe that the clinical material of this session offers some interesting food for thought on the fundamental characteristics of my patient's personality. Let's begin with his thoughts on physical height. In the first instance, it would seem that Al simply expresses the desire to become tall like me, or superior to me, in order to escape the danger of being called a "shrimp", looked down upon, considered to be inferior. This is probably true, but only partly, because after a while it turns out that his real worry is that his plans to grow have not been completed according to the timetable he had set out for it, despite the pains he had taken to drink so much milk, present in his ice-creams, and in doing sport so he could stand up straighter. He can't stand it when things haven't gone "exactly" as he predicted, two centimetres in July, two in August, two in September. And now the measure of his height is not exactly how I had calculated on the schedule. The preciseness of his calculations is put under discussion about the measuring stick's evidence. Only with great difficulty do I manage to convince him he is wrong. In the end I am firmly compelled to ask him to trust the "objective measuring stick", without, as a result, having to renounce the idea of being able to grow taller than me. I encourage him not to flee from reality, inventing a height that is not in fact his, or transforming the negative result into an apocalyptic disaster.

The firmness of the tone of my voice at this point pushes him to "tidy up" his pockets and to abandon himself to an apparently more constructive attitude. He makes sure I understand that he knows special words like "indigo", that he knows how to clearly enunciate or sing, and what's more, he knows how to speak in a "countrified" manner. In the attempt to astonish me or to joke around, he instead becomes immediately repetitive until it's exhausting, at which point I have to stop him again, telling him that he is a pain in the bottom.

This produces a new change which makes him confront both his ignorance and my own, when faced with rainbows. At this point, he surprisingly shows a capacity to tolerate of not knowing the answer, an ability he did not possess when he was a child. What allows us to understand how his impulse is to avoid these two experiences is linked to a particular vision of the word in which life is a game where you can win prizes, where even the loss of the second session and the end of his therapy are considered much in the same way as an elimination from the game. At this point a sudden transformation takes place in his body, beyond his control: a cold suddenly "explodes" in him, activating the production of abundant mucus, which "blocks" him.

The acts of opening oneself up to emotional reality, to searching for the reasons behind feelings, remaining in ignorance, in uncertainty, is perhaps still too difficult for Al. It is an experience which he cannot tolerate because on one hand it leaves him defenceless, forcing him to acutely feel *uselessness and failure* in his efforts to be tall enough; on the other hand, it fills him with *too many questions*, to which he does not know how to find an answer, also because his symbolic processes and his vocabulary are not good enough, as evidenced by his use of the word "elimination" to speak of a loss. All that is left for him is to free himself, at the earliest opportunity, from the physical discomfort of his blocked nose, and also to compensate his blocked ears, caused by blowing hard into the tissue. Apparently he is successful. I notice that his mucus stops flowing in the same sudden way as it had appeared.

From this moment on, Al is struggling with phenomena not as easily measurable as are our bodily heights, which we can determine with the stick. These phenomena are linked to the light and to the images, which it leaves on the walls of the room, and also to the self-hypnotic current which sends us to sleep, and to the permanence of bodily warmth left on objects. Is he perhaps trying to understand or to discover how memories are born, how images from a past can be seen again or how one can imagine something that does not yet exist? At this point it might be useful to think that the initial theme of the "physical height" could figure out an attempt on Al's part to reflect on the emotional and mental growth to which he would like to apply an exact "metre", whilst discovering that every small step towards the world of meanings brings with it the danger of confusion, of ignorance and of the mystery of the existence of something which cannot be reduced to the world of sensations and perceptions, of measurable things: *it transports him into a world which is too crowded of questions*. At the end of the session, he seems to wonder how it could be possible that what disappears and becomes unfathomable can persist in the memory, that what is intangible takes form on a mental screen like the shadows on the walls of the therapy room.

Alessio (fifteen years and seven months)

Al arrives on time. He quickly says hello to me, with a slightly reverential bow and then, after asking for permission, he goes to the bathroom and then returns to the therapy room. I cannot follow him immediately, because his mother stops me in the corridor to pay for the previous month's sessions, and to ask me if her son had spoken to me about the sudden death of S, his favourite uncle. When I tell her that he hadn't, she tells me that it had seemed to her for a while that his son has become a "philosopher", since he is so indifferent to the deaths of a few people he was very close to, such as his grandfather and his uncle S. I think inwardly about how Al is dealing with the end of the therapy sessions, and in light of everything I am observing, I think that it is too harsh to define his behaviour as "indifferent". I believe, on the contrary, that his being a "philosopher" is his own special way of coming to terms with the loss of people and things dear to him.

I finally join him in the therapy room. He immediately wants to know what I was talking about with his mother. I explain to him, but he doesn't seem to want to stop what he is doing in order to speak about the death of his uncle. He has a piece of paper in front of him on which he had drawn in capital and in bold near the end of one of our previous sessions, the word "TRE" (three) with an arrow which pointed to the number three, and the three capital letters XRS. During that session he had made a confused reference to the opening theme tune of one of RAI 3's programmes. He is using his pencil to put extra touches to the letter "S", which looked slightly wonky, because of the conspicuous font he had chosen for it (the "S" did not seem to be able to stand upright, and gave the impression of falling on one side). He is also writing in bold a name, which corresponds to each letter: xylophone, radio, spring.

He notices that he does not have enough room underneath to be able to write all three words and so he starts a major task of copying and pasting. He cuts the blank bit off the top of the paper and goes to add it underneath with a piece of adhesive tape. He is very much absorbed in his work. I stay silent, also because I have learnt from previous experience that he would not listen if I spoke now. After a few minutes of silence, he suddenly lifts his head and, looking me straight in the eyes, asks whether I am his mother's boss. He goes back to his work. I would like to explore the meaning of his question with him, but I am aware that my request for clarification has more to do with my need to tackle my astonishment, which makes it really necessary to get some sort of explanation out of him. I think of Al who, as a small child, would say to his mother who called from the publicity office where she worked: "Mum, why 'I am' crying?" and of the period of therapy sessions in which he would, for weeks, start to draw maps, telling me that he was a "designer".

I decide, in any case, to use this sudden break of the silence to repeat to him what I had told him in the last two sessions, regarding the number three and the letters TRE on his "poster". The three makes me think of the number of weekly sessions of therapy work, which he had undergone for so many years, which was now about to come to an end. He makes me repeat all this because he had decided not to listen to me. I repeat. He stands up and tells me affirmatively that the time has really come for him to finish, since he's been coming to these sessions for a long time. Then he approaches my chair to ask me if, without my help, he will be capable in future of managing his "bad behaviour". I tell him that I don't know, and I add that, if he ever found himself in difficulty, I will always be here for him to come and talk to.

He sits back down at the table to finish his endeavour of sticking the pieces of paper together. Then he starts to repeatedly and slowly move the sheet up and down, the words in front of his eyes, until they disappear behind his head. I ask him what this gesture means. He gets up and approaches me. He starts to make the sheet go up and down in front of my eyes, and demonstrates as such that the action has something to do with the scrolling of film clips. Then he goes to the window and, whilst looking out of it, he tells me about a television programme in which there is an actor who, when making a similar gesture to that which he himself has just made with the sheet, says "how handsome I am!" just when his face is revealed. So I remind him that a long time ago he also used to often go into the bathroom to look in the mirror, saying "gorgeous creature!" at his own reflection. I tell him that I think that there is a small child in him, who for months felt like a "gorgeous creature" whenever he was reflected in the eyes of his mother, but when this same child, from the moment in which he was weaned, felt that he was no longer a beautiful and beloved child. I suggest to him that perhaps all this has something to do with how he feels about our goodbye.

At this point Al, in his characteristic way, latches onto the word "goodbye" and starts to talk to me about the contemptuous and enraged goodbye with which Marisa, the beautiful and prosperous lady from the Marche region, leaves Marino, the barber from Ciociaria, in Latium, in the film *Straziami ma di baci saziami* (Torture Me But Fill Me up with Kisses). She leaves her beloved because she believes he has cheated on her with the "harlot Adelaide". He also talks of the tormented and painful goodbye between doctor Zhivago and Lara, whose drama returns in the same film, at the same moment in which Marisa and Marino, still in love but their passion opposed by her father, decide to die together, jumping in front of a train. He recites the scenes from the two films off by heart, he acts out the characters, and he softly sings the soundtrack of Lara's theme. He amuses himself replicating Marisa's "countrified" accent, repeating again his bad words and insults towards Marino, but above all he repeats a phrase that Marisa says to Marino: "If I were you I would be ashamed", or tries to take on, less successfully, the melodramatic and romantic air of the doctor Zhivago. I humour his dramatization of these two goodbyes for a while; they are actually quite playful and entertaining. Then I suggest that perhaps the opposing feelings, which come along with the two experiences of separation, portrayed in the two scenes of the film are present in his relationship with me, now that we are coming to the end of the therapy sessions.

Whilst I am talking to him, Al stops his narrative and seizes the calendar, flicking through it until he finds the month of May. He marks off all the past days with a cross, but avoids doing the same for today's date, May 9th. It seems as though he wants to keep from crossing the 9th off until he reaches the end of the session. At this point, he starts to cut out (he says "carve") with the scissors a piece of white rectangular paper. He does so with maximum precision. He tells me that he is preparing a fax, which he will use to transcribe a message to his father, which he heard, before coming to the session, on the house answerphone. I remind him of his furious and regretful reaction to the past ban which I had imposed on him (for reasons of privacy) from listening to recorded messages on the answerphone in my waiting room, and I ask him whether his father would really be happy that he is listening to messages on the house answerphone, with the risk of deleting them. He tells me that he wants to bring the sheet to the house, to transcribe the message that he heard. Just as the hour comes to an end, the doorbell rings. It is his father, who has come to pick him up.

Al, spontaneously, starts to tidy up his things in the box and, mostly to create a bit of orderliness, to throw the useless bits of paper, which are sitting on the table into the bin, instead of keeping them. In throwing away the waste paper, he pretends it is a basketball hoop, and throws the paper in from far away. He gets it in first time, and looks at me with great satisfaction. He picks up his mobile and the paper tissues, which he had placed on the table at the beginning of the session. He puts them in his pocket next to the fax, and also pockets the adhesive tape. I point this out to him. "Ooops!" he says, and puts it back into the box. Then he notices the calendar and quickly, with a blue felt-tip, crosses out the 9th May. Then he closes the lid of the box, and leaves the therapy room calmly. He reaches his father who is waiting for him, smiling, before the office's exit at the end of the corridor. Al does not greet him. He seems to be in a hurry to get home to transcribe the answerphone message. They leave the office together. Less than five minutes later the doorbell rings and Al is back again, who wanted to give me back the blue felt-tip which he had taken away without my noticing.

Commentary

In the course of his therapy Al has rarely felt so calm, and at the same time so ready to step out from his usual script, to look for a meeting point with me and to take care of his things, as he has in this session. Consequently I have rarely felt such a deep pleasure in being with him. What is the secret behind all this?

I think that the answer can be found in the fact that today he is self-confident and feels sure that he can leave his mark on people and on things; as he said, he has become a good sculptor, he has learned to "carve", he feels that what belongs to him also has a relevance to me, like the bold type and numbers which he draws on the sheet. At the same time he accepts that I am putting my script first, in which I focus on the theme of the end of the therapy, on our goodbye, and because of this he seems to appreciate the value of some instruments, like the calendar, which I made available to help him consider the passing of time.

Moreover, I believe that the brief meeting I had with his mother at the beginning of the session is important. It is an episode, which evocatively illustrates how his mother's depression could have influenced the characteristics of his internal world. As she had done in our very first meeting, she speaks of her son as being "in a bubble", this time in a bubble of indifference about the deaths of his grandfather and of his uncle, two people to whom he was very close. Astonished and confused about his "philosophical" behaviour, she seems to wonder why her son is so "naughty". Her own depression pushes her to be very severe and bitter towards him, to take on a reproachful attitude towards him.

I know from experience that children like Al are capable of experiencing very intense feelings about the death of someone close to them, but only when they relive the same positive feelings of dependence in a new relationship (sometimes an analytical one), that they had felt for a loved one in the past. Months or years can go by before this happens. I maintain, then, that it is wrong to consider and judge them "indifferent" and "naughty" because their actions do not live up to our expectations (seeing them cry at the funeral, seeing them need more closeness).

Al could also appear indifferent about the end of the therapy. In fact, he has declared more often during these last sessions "I don't give a toss about Dr B", but he says this, looking me directly in the face and speaking in a "countrified" way (like Marisa jokingly does in the film *Torture Me But Fill Me up with Kisses*). I feel it is vital that he can "attack" with his indifference—rage, as if this was *his way to get inside me and at the same time get me to live inside him*. I am convinced that as the years go by Al fully shares our "humanity". There has been no evidence which makes me doubt that he is able to experience our same emotions, anguish and fear; that he does not think about life and death, as the rest of us do; that he is not interested in understanding the difference between things we can see and things we cannot see; that he does not wonder why people and things which are now here can disappear; that he does not ask himself what is that thing which we call "soul", where we come from, who we are born from; that he is completely incapable of seeing himself in the future, of having expectations of himself and of other people. I am instead convinced that his "otherness" is irreducibly linked to his own particular way of organising what is our common "humanity". We see in the material from this session, (and above all the next session), that the introjective processes, which are at the base of the main characteristics of his internal world, function, at this point of his symbolic development, differently from our own. This partly would explain the compulsiveness and immaturity of his thought and his preference to still live in a "bubble".

In this regard it is possible to pinpoint the mental mechanisms, which Al uses to give permanency, consistency to things and to people and to remember them, removing them from the flow of time. His approach has something to do with "sculpting" the object of his interest, which vary in underlining, framing, imitating, highlighting with a cross; it also has something to do with finding once more the object of his interest, flicking the film clips of reality incessantly backwards and forwards. This session and the following are good examples of how the game of *"Bu-Bu settete"* (the Italian version of "peek-a-boo") is born, and demonstrate how there can only be a surprise if the object lingers in the memory during its absence: and that the loss of someone cannot be felt if this person does not live concretely inside us. How can we make a person live inside us if we are missing perspective as a symbolic form? If we are missing an internal world we can place it in? The object is, then, followed in its passage like a planet which crosses our line of vision and, as such, takes form, becomes three-dimensional, only sculpting it, with the help of the light which shows up its features, making it stand out from the backdrop.

I would now like to present you with the material of the following session, in which it is possible to clearly see this continuous oscillation of approaching and moving away from symbolic thought.

Alessio (fifteen years and seven months)

He is slightly late. I hear him "calling" the lift; he speaks to it as though he wanted to make it arrive earlier, more quickly. On the threshold of the office door he greets me, with a reverential bow, telling me "*Buon Gorno*". I notice he intentionally leaves out the "i" from "Buongiorno". I tell him that today he might well joke around, in order to be forgiven for his slight lateness to the session. He heads towards the therapy room. He stops for a while on the threshold, playing with the light switch. Now his behaviour seems less playful. He seems to want to irritate me. He looks at the ceiling light, which is going on and off, and comments "artificial light". Then he comes into the room, heading straight for the window, which opens onto a luminous garden, and he speaks to me of "sunlight". I think that he is perhaps hoping to be forgiven for something, maybe something which relates to one of his aggressive actions in the past, when in the winter season on more than one occasion he had insisted on turning the light off in the room, telling me that it was "good like this", succeeding in sending us into a blacker darkness, as the evening approached little by little. At the same time in this little skirmish, I understand his major desire to be "a protagonist", not to be blocked by me.

He goes to sit down on the seat, and pulls the calendar out of the box. With the blue felt-tip he marks a cross on every day of the week since I last saw him, and leaves crossing off today's date, the 6th, for the end of the hour. He flicks through the calendar (it is big, and in book form, with a picture and a photograph for each month of the year that captures the passing of seasons). He stops to read the caption of the month of January, which is dedicated to a photograph of Aprica, a locality in the mountains of Northern Italy. There is lots of snow. He tells me that "Aprica" makes him think of "Africa". He again seems to want to joke around, transforming words by changing letters at his whim, the "p" to an "f". I don't say anything to him because in the meantime he has started to slide the blue marker across his face, as he had done in the previous session with the sheet on which he had written the television logo "three" in capitals. I notice that he does move his eyes to follow the movement of the object: he moves the marker repeatedly in his line of vision, first to one side, then coming out of the other as if he were filming a scene with a fixed camera, to accentuate the idea of an empty space which fills up and then empties again. Speaking to him of the fact that at the end of the last session he took away the blue marker, I tell him that perhaps he is, deep down, searching for something which would enable him to take away something that he could look at again, like a film which could remind him of my presence and of his box.

Al wants to know the exact date of the last session. Looking at the calendar together, we establish that the last session will be Monday 11th July, because he will, as usual, leave for a holiday at the seaside with his relatives during the second half of the month. He draws a little sign next to the date, underlining it, he says, to remember it and remind him not to cross it off. Then he begins to joke around again, saying again and again "I don't give a toss about Dr B". I tell him again that he really likes to joke about the separation but I know that his "not giving a toss" is not his real feeling, or at least not all of his sentiments. He stops joking around. He firmly closes the pages of the calendar, putting one, which is sticking out back in. He does it with the same placidity and rhythm of voice with which I had spoken to him. He points out to me that in the photograph of May there is no more snow that it has disappeared. He is thinking of something, which is changing, disappearing, it melts like snow, of a transformation.

Then, as he puts the calendar back with his toys, he starts to speak of the weather. He insists that I tell him what the weather will be like tomorrow, in a week, what the weather was like in May last year. He looks out of the window and notes that the weather is grey. He stands up, approaches me and, looking insistently at me, subjects me to an exhausting and pressing interrogation in which he wants to know when the sky will be clear or when there will be mist. I try to extract myself from his thousands of questions, repeating to him that I am not a weatherman and that he is more of an expert on these things than I am, then that we are not wizards who can say for certain what the weather will be like in future. He starts to pace up and down the room, discoursing or interrogating me on the weather forecasts. He goes more and more often to the window to look at what the weather is doing. He seems to want to check if the weather is stable or if the greyness will soon give way to a sunny sky.

Now he seems to be interested in the mist. Whilst he is trying to explain to me what mist is, he almost unwittingly stops close to me and starts to tidy me up quite carefully, smoothing the folds of my shirt collar, placing my woollen jumper under the collar, as if he wanted to cover me better, make me feel warmer (I am feeling a lot of tenderness, when on other occasions his same actions distance me from him). His actions resemble those of a mother who rearranges her child's clothes, before sending him out into the open, where it is cold. Then he sits down on the couch, before adjusting the coloured throw on top of it, then he starts to lightly scratch away at the places where he seems to see bits of dirt (maybe invisible bits of play-dough).

Quite gradually I feel that today I am not alone in fighting against the large and chaotic cloud of his questions and of his pseudoscientific interests. If Al is not really ready to give me back my freedom today he at least seems ready to let me avoid his insolence, out of his pressing need to come back with "exact" answers, certain forecasts. In the end I tell him that I don't specialise in the weather, but in how he is feeling, in the "weather" there is inside him.

Whilst I am speaking to him in this trivial way, I notice that from this complex moment of interaction onwards (I inwardly think of the Bionian "cloud"), an element starts to emerge, the mist, which seems to create a bridge between our two minds. From this moment we begin to speak of mist and we carry on at length like this, sharing our ideas on the relationship between the sun and the light, on the fact that mist is an impalpable thing which light goes through, which allows one to see objects and at the same time hides them from view. He mimes going through a sheet of mist with his body, or emerging from something visible but impalpable and associates the mist with ghosts.

He starts speaking to me about Casper, the good and gentle ghost of an adolescent who lives in Whipstaff's castle in the small town of Friendship, in Maine, in the company of three cunning uncles with strange and provocative names, Fatso, Stinkie, and Stretch, where the doctor Harvey arrives at a certain point. He is a psychoanalyst who specialises in ghosts, and has a daughter, Kat, with whom Casper falls in love.

Al emphasises the benefits of being a ghost, "you are immortal [in the past he told me I was a member of the immortals, the Highlanders], you never get ill, you can never be injured, captured, you can go through walls". I remind him that in the film the two lovers Casper and Kat suffer from loneliness because their essences are so different that they cannot fulfil their love. In a crescendo, he tells me about the machine that can create ghosts, the potion which makes you go back to being human again, and about souls and about ghosts created with a computer which exist only in the electronic bit; he tells me about Halloween.

I feel dazed and overwhelmed with all of this information he is throwing at me. Not to become his victim, I try to meticulously go over the conversation word for word, to try and shed some light on a few connections, to better complete or arrange some scenes, to clarify the plot of the film. I again feel as though I were being tossed around in a cloud made of diffused, fragmented, scattered particles. As if I had heard something incoherent from which a story could be born, or had helped with the incessant hammer and chisel work of marble sculptor without yet knowing what his model was.

At this point he stops for a second to ask me a precise question. Incredulous and fearful, he wants to know whether ghosts really exist, and asks me whether they are hidden in the walls. When waiting for my reply, he looks at the walls and touches them as if he wanted to find some confirmation or denial of his worries. At this point I tell him that perhaps he is asking who invented ghosts and why they exist. I tell him, arousing his interest, that often young children, when they are frightened by a sudden loud noise, are made to think "that it was a ghost", and even primitive men (during this time he had spoken to me of the Australopithecus), who didn't know the nature of natural extreme and dangerous phenomena thought, for example, that a lightning bolt was hurled at the earth by a ghostly god, who was hidden behind the clouds. I thus speak to him of "ghosts" as a product of our minds, of our imagination, as a name which we use to evoke something violent and dangerous, of which we do not know the cause, we do not see the origin, but unleashes a strong reaction of fear in us.

He calms down and starts to look at his image reflected in the windowpane. He tells me that his image is his ghost (his soul?), which wants to get in the room, to get inside of him. I succeed only in telling him that his shadow is something true, whilst ghosts are a product of his imagination. I get the feeling that he is preparing a new cloud of confusion. Unfortunately the hour is over. I tell him so. I feel exhausted. He stops for a moment to cross out today's date with the blue felt-tip. Then, before closing the calendar and putting it in the box, he runs the palm of his hand across the days already crossed off, as if he wanted to caress them or to capture them to take away with him.

Commentary

Many of Al's actions in this session deserve to be marked out because of their relevance to our discussion: the desire to joke around (sometimes amusingly, sometimes annoyingly), the intense activity with his hands and with his eyes (sometimes labouring in the work of a sculptor, sometimes magic in the work of a wizard apprentice) and his interests in natural phenomena (sometimes genuine, sometimes pseudoscientific).

It could be said that these activities and interests have been present in the therapeutic practice since the very first session. They prevalently belong to three different relationships that originally belong to his actual life: firstly, with his dead grandfather, a playful and highly patient person who loved to do fun things such as taking him to play on the merry-go-round or going to a restaurant together; secondly, with his mother, creative by profession, who relaxes with embroidery; thirdly, with his researcher father, with whom he often spends the weekends in a country home.

At the same time, a great change can be observed: Al, despite being deeply shaped by these relationships, has for years been tackling a new and complex relational experience, a therapeutic one, which, because of its length, has become a new and important chapter in his personal life. His psychoanalyst has become an expert in "ghosts", in "souls", in mists, in reflective and projective surfaces, in lights and shadows, which capture his interest in what is behind things. He has always incited him to move towards the immaterial, keeping him in the world of "questions" with his profound outlook on the reality of the mind, in the hope that this will help him to discover his subjectivity, to really know himself.

Alessio (fifteen years and nine months): penultimate session

It is summer. He arrives late. With a gloomy face he makes me understand that he is beside himself, angry with his mother who, to punish him for his being late, has threatened not to take him to the seaside any longer. He is thinking about killing her, throwing big stones against her, or about doing himself in, killing himself, jumping out of the window. He opens the window and looks at the garden below. I go near him, to try to calm him down. I tell him that it cannot be true that his mother has decided to prevent him from doing the things that he likes, like going to the seaside. I point out that his mother is right to be angry with him because he often happens not to be ready when it is time to go out for an appointment either with me or at school. I tell him that his mother seems to be fed up with this kind of behaviour, because she is very tired, especially now that grandfather is no longer there to help her out. I invite him to think that sometimes his mother is so aggrieved that she tells him nasty things that she will never carry out. He replies that he has not thought about that. In any case, he is very doubtful that his mother is willing to forgive him. "Only if I'm lucky", he says to me.

Keeping in mind the only dream that he has brought to therapy so far, in which his mother slapped him, I talk to him about how easily he feels his mother's threats to punish him as something terrible, just as he experienced as "hellish" the scolding of his father and of his uncle when he was a child. I suggest that perhaps he feels like that because of the guilt he experiences when his parents make him feel "all wrong", someone to get rid of, like bad, stinky poo. He replies that guilt is disgusting. I then tell him that it is important to be able to acknowledge that he was wrong, and that if he apologises to his mother for having been late today and is then punished less harshly than she had anticipated, he will see that everything will be alright. He replies that he does not believe it, and I should be the one to tell his mother this. I suggest he should do this himself and let me intervene only if things do not go well with his mother. I also remark that many if these clashes take place with his mother because he is not independent, he is not free to make his own choices and then confront me or his teachers directly. For this, I tell him that he is very good at hiding behind his mother's back.

I ask him: "Today, for example, why were you not ready so as to arrive to your session on time?" Bluntly, he replies: "These are private matters."

In a playful tone of voice, referring to a specific game, which had kept him occupied for months when he was a child, I tell him that the ones in charge today are the little red light men, those who raise the signs that say "no entry". He tries to be a bit standoffish. In the box, he finds the signs that say "no entry" and "all clear" (there are more than one); with a rather harsh expression, as if to tell me that I'll never have it my own way, he repeats his game many times, putting himself in the shoes of the tyrant. I joke about his refusal to tell me about the reasons for having been late, saying that now I am the child who deserves to be punished, while he has become the bad mother who wants to get rid of me because he-she is irritated by the stubbornness with which I keep demanding something from him.

He interrupts my comments to show me that on the back of a sheet there are three capital letters, ATR, within a circle. He cannot tell me what their meaning might be, and I suggest that maybe A stands for Al, R for Roberto, my name, but I do not know about T. After a moment of silence he tells me that T is for "Testa" (head). My interpretation is that it is true: despite so many "no entry" areas, Doctor B and Al have been able to spend many years together to think, use their heads and try to understand the difference that one makes when one "uses his head" and thinks, instead of being carried away by anger and fear, or by farts and magic spells. I tell him that, at least in part, we have managed to do that, even if there are still some moments in which I notice how difficult it is for him to keep his behaviour under control and understand the meaning of that, like when, for example, he is not ready to go out for an appointment or when he finds something else to do at the very last moment, a bit like what happens at the end of our therapy sessions, when he must leave my office. In conclusion, I tell him that there is something that we need to understand about his being such a "Mr Wobbly". He asks me what I mean by "wobbly", and I explain the meaning of the word to him. I remind him that when he was a child I often talked about his infantile parts using a language that I had borrowed from some English books for children (he does not remember), whose characters were called Mr Jelly, Mr No and also Mr Rabbit.

He immediately remembers the film about *Roger Rabbit* and names the director and the main character. Films are his passion; he often uses his knowledge of cinema to show me how many things he knows that I am ignorant of. Then he stands up and starts playing "catch the witch", an old game whose contents and associations have never been very clear to me.

He isolates himself. Exactly as he did when he was little, he starts making his fingers "fly" as if they were two imaginary witches that precipitously fell after suddenly losing their nature of magical creatures or after being thrown off their flying broomsticks by a spiteful, powerful wizard. I ask him, unsuccessfully, to make me understand what he is doing with his hands, but he does not hear me and starts walking up and down the room a couple of times, always playing with his hands, making the witches fly and fall. Then he stops in front of the window and starts walking, moving a single leg, as if he had a cramp. He pretends to be lame, explaining to me that he also used to do that when he was little. He laughs, amused by his own performance.

Then, suddenly, he becomes gloomy. Again, he is thinking about the punishment that his mother anticipated for his being late. He opens the window and threatens to jump off. I move near him and I stand with my back to the window ledge; I look him in the eye and once again I ask him to tell me why today, as usual, he was not prepared to come. He explains to me that just before leaving home he started washing his feet, because "they stank" (a stench from Hell).

I remind him that quite often, in the past, he left my room late at the end of the session because he would spend a long time washing his hands, his "willie" and even his feet in the bidet, once or twice. My interpretation is that perhaps today he is telling me that he is not ready to leave his therapy, that he is not able to think what it means to say goodbye forever; he is unable to make his head work, because "stink" captures his whole attention. "What is this stink all about—I ask him—that you do not want me to smell, that you want to keep hidden from everybody?"

He sits down and raises the "all clear" sign. Then he takes the July calendar, the printed one, and watches it carefully. I remind him that there is only one session left before the end of therapy, before our final goodbye. I notice that, for a moment, his gaze becomes rather sad (in the past, snot would come out of his nose). Then, as if wanting not to be sad, he places the calendar on the table, stands up and starts speechifying: he repeatedly says that his mother is a "sinner" and that she deserves to be punished. Again, he expresses his wish to stone her to death. I repeat what I told him at the beginning of the session, namely that he cannot have faith in my suggestion to apologise to his mother for what happened and to tell her that he is ready to accept a less severe punishment than the one she promised him. I talk to him as I stand up in front of the window. He repeats that my duty is to act as an ambassador to his mother, also because my proposal is too long. When I refuse, he slowly slides down on the floor, lying there and pretending to be dead. He keeps his eyes closed and remains motionless for a few minutes. I tell him that he is showing me how complicated things can get when one is unable to keep a mother/witch out of one's mind, becoming incapable of thinking at all. Then, the relationship with his mother turns into an all-out war, full of hatred and extortions, in which he tries to hit her and instil fear in her, frightening her with his threat to kill himself, or pretending to be dead. The same thing happens when he feels the need to take away the stink from his body, becoming incapable of thinking.

Our time is up; he goes to the bathroom to drink and wash his hands. He leaves the door open and, consequently, he hears all that I am saying to his mother, who seems to accept the idea that her son's "being late" might be related to his resistance to coming to the sessions because the end is approaching. We also agree on Al's need to learn to be a bit more independent. I do not hint, on purpose, to the proposal I discussed with him in the session. Al comes out of the bathroom and vehemently asks, orders his mother to take him to the seaside. Instead of containing him, the mother becomes confused and tells him that they cannot go to the seaside because the seawater is "polluted" by salmonella. Al does not understand this, becomes angrier and threatens to hit her. She makes me notice her son's "animosity" and tells me that this way of reacting has lately become worse, together with the tendency to lie or to pretend to listen.

While his mother is going downstairs, I stop Al for a second, to give me a proper goodbye. He stops, turns around, stares at my eyes and squeezes my arms tightly, conveying to me all his anger towards a mother who, "in his opinion", is very bad and unable to understand him. In a low voice, I encourage him to keep calm, and to tell his mother what I suggested, feeling certain that in this way everything will be alright, and that his mother will forgive him.

Commentary

Also in this session, like in the previous one, emerges the theme of *perfection*, this time in terms of moral judgement, and not in terms of knowledge. The *"mischief"* (being late) replaces the *"wrong answer"*. Thus, what changes is the geography, the stage where Al's infantile drama unfolds, and the consequences are therefore different: from the TV studio, where the wrong answer forces you to leave the game, now he has moved inside the Sistine Chapel, above or below, in Heaven or in Hell, two opposite extremes. A religious vision is juxtaposed to the real experience, making the conflict between the infantile Self and its object unsolvable if not by means of capital punishment or the request of indulgent forgiveness. Once again, I make an effort to distance Al from the unavoidability of this view of the world, showing him how the two "extremes"—his own, who angrily fights against injustice, and his mother's, who has punished him—are the diseased fruit of a primary confusion between good and bad, and of the difficulty in believing that things can be repaired by understanding their emotional meaning.

I wonder whether his hatred for the punishment may also have something to do with his mother's decision to interrupt the therapy, which appears to him as a prematurely induced birth, with nobody there to welcome him, or simply as an incomprehensible surrender.

Alessio: final session

He arrives on time. He takes the lift. He has a closed umbrella with him. Outside, the weather is threatening rain. As soon as he sees me he starts to play the "23 game", a sort of "eenie meenie miny moe" game with the steps, and says "what an ass", which makes him laugh a lot.

He repeats a game originally linked to an experiment with his maternal grandfather who had, when he was little, taught him the names of each of the fingers: thumb, index finger, middle finger, ring finger, and little finger. But once, when he was irritated by his grandson's infinite requests to repeat the game, he lost it and added onto the end of the usual sequence a liberating "what an ass". Al had then interpreted the "what an ass" to be the name of another finger.

At the same time he looks at me, measuring my height. I say nothing until we are both sitting in the therapy room. He opens the box, which is on the table, and looks at the calendar—whilst I remind him that this is the last session, the goodbye. "Oh yes", he comments, hiding a little behind the box. Straight after, he adds: "Well it can really be said then that I don't give a toss about doctor B!" and that "now with the break, the holidays are coming, which are important". I tell him that his claims don't match up to his true feelings. And he answers: "Yep, it's a joke." I remind him again that today's is really the last session, and I talk to him about how much time has passed since our very first meeting, when he was still in nursery school ("I was a nursed-type", he jokes). I comment that today he is a man, who isn't a little boy anymore and who has "learned to use his head", to be himself. He gets angry and points out that he has always been himself.

Then he starts to pick up some sheets and colours because he wants to draw the calendar of July, the month of the year we are currently in. He shows me the calendar, which he drew in February. He looks at it and comments: "It's perfect". Then he starts a detailed analysis on the "absolute" perfection of God, and the "imperfection" of us humans. He explains to be that only in Heaven can we enjoy the perfection of God. Then with a priestly air, he tells me that Gaius and Brutus, who killed Caesar, are "evil" and certainly ended up in Hell, where a burning stench comes from.

I remind him that he also turned up to the last session full of "furious" and "homicidal" feelings towards his mother, seemingly wanting to crush her by throwing rocks at her. His mother became a witch-mother in his mind when, to punish him for his continual lateness, had threatened to no longer take him to the seaside. I invite him not to fall into his usual mistake of "simplifying things" and I tell him that no one, above all his mother, has ever thought of sending him to Hell. I tell him that this perfect God, who, he is speaking to me about and which demands so much perfection, is a God which has maybe forgotten about humankind, and that perhaps only love can close the gap that exists between God and humankind.

I add that I am talking to him about his idea of perfection, about his desire to be perfect, so perfect that it isolates him from everyone else, stopping him from getting closer to people, with the outcome that having achieved his desired perfection, he would find himself completely alone. He gets up from the chair and approaches me with the little scissors and tells me that he is going to use them, after having finished the calendar, to cut out a trumpet, like the ones on those old gramophones, to use to stick on his recording device, which will amplify the sounds and help him to hear the recorded voices better.

He starts to make the calendar of July. In a silent pause, when I am sure that I will not distract him and make him make a mistake when he is bustling about with his colours, I ask him how it has been with his mother, if his mother has forgiven him or not (today he arrived on time). He answers positively, in the tone of someone who is thinking "Of course!" Then, lifting his eyes to me, he confesses that "he has really been very lucky", as if to tell me that I was right to maintain that his mother was not an evil witch who should be stoned, but that I had been "really very lucky" in my guess that, if he apologised to her, everything would go back to normal. He seems to tell me that I have been good and "lucky", like those who answer correctly on television game shows.

He gets back to his creation of the July calendar. He shows me a letter "S" from "Saturday", and asks whether it is comprehensible. I joke around, telling him that the "S" looks a bit tired, slanting, as if it needed to have to lie down on some cushions (he can never do an "S" properly). He smiles, amused, and seems contented with how it has come out. I think that "S" is the initial of his dead uncle's name. At other times, he would have torn the sheet into small pieces and thrown it in the bin. At a certain point, he realises that one sheet is not enough to write all the days of July, and that he needs to add another one to it. He quickly solves the problem with a cutting and pasting task, which allows him the space, which he needs to finish writing all the days on the calendar. He then crosses out the dates of our past sessions, and gives me the calendar, telling me to use it to cross out the dates which would have been our sessions over the coming weeks. In the meantime I speak to him about the importance that the calendar has had in our work. I point out that at the start of the therapy, it had been me to create it, which, as a child, had really interested and surprised him, but also provoked feelings of inferiority and a lot of anger.

I remind him that at that time he also thought I was Doc from *Back to the Future*, whereas now he is creating the calendar all by himself; he concentrates so he does not make a mistake, he toils and repairs without magic, and moreover, is happy to give me the last one he made as a gift, so I could take it away as a memory. He listens to me. Then, suddenly, he starts ask himself, and also indirectly to ask me, whether it is more correct to say "Bu-Bu settete" or "Bu-Bu sette" (the name of a television programme). He then begins to play a game of "Bu-Bu settete", which he translates in English as "Seven-se!" I feel lost. I fear I have lost him. Instead, he starts to explain to me that he uses the "Bu-Bu settete" with the added "te" to convey "surprise", giving me the example of the gesture one makes when getting out of water. He explains then that he uses "Bu-Bu sette", without the final "te", when he wants to convey "exactness", to affirm that his answer is exact, the right one, just like when he is on a train or in a car, and he correctly guesses the name of the next station or small town. He asks me how it gets to be like this.

I talk to him about the onomatopoeic sound of the "te" at the end of "Bu-bu sette", giving him the example of the noise that knuckles make against a door, which can frighten but also signal the presence of something interesting, of someone to whom it is perhaps worth paying attention. I add that in this "te", there may be the whole experience that we have had together, like when he was little and was surprised to see my calendar for the first time, and started to become aware of me.

I think to myself that through the therapeutic experience he may have internalised, the difference between experiencing an emotion together with someone else (a "te"/"you") and the excitement of perfection, between the "Bu-Bu settete" and the Bu-Bu sette.

I have to tell him that time has run out, that the session is over. Before I let him leave, I express my appreciation for his diligence and for the effort he has put in today to "use his head to think". He leaves the room and goes straight to the bathroom, where he urinates and then flushes the toilet. He moves to the sink, where he washes his face and hands several times. He drinks a few sips from the tap. Then lightly pushing the tap up and down, he plays at modulating the water pressure, which is coming out of the flush (as a child he was terrified of the sound of the flush). Having finished this concert, he leaves the bathroom and repeatedly plays at catching the air in the corridor, putting it into his mouth with his fist and pretending to swallow it. He takes in the silicon dust in the air, those little particles that can only be seen very close against the light. This is his way of parting when it is time to go home, his way of saying "bye".

Then he asks me if he can go back in the room because he wants to make the trumpet to attach to his recording device to amplify the sound. I tell him that the time is up, but if he likes, he can take a blank piece of paper to take home, where he can take his time doing whatever he likes. He finally leaves the office. He disappears onto the landing without saying goodbye. His head is already elsewhere.

Commentary

The theme of "perfection" is back once more, this time in the world of emotions and thought. Al seems to think that there are two types of perfection which he is always looking for: an old one, where he must find the right answer, and a new one, the discovery that it is possible to find a correspondence, a congruity, a resonance in someone or in something outside of oneself; the discovery of the "te" ("you") in the "Bu-Bu settete", which, like a birth (as the image of the person coming out of the sea suggests) captures the soul of whoever achieves it, or of the person who is observing it and making the experience of sharing personal emotions possible.

Discussion

Being told that he is good, handsome and kind is something that every child normally expects from him relatives. Managing to hear that he is made of good stuff, that he is a "gorgeous creature", that he is up to a task, is the foundation of one's childlike self. With the pervasive impediments to his development, including his autism, all of this trade in sentiments never gets off the ground, or happens late, or only partly happens, and the child grows up with a very scarce knowledge of the self and of the people who are surrounding him, with an inconsistent "Ego" and inadequate internal objects.

In the introduction I expressed the certainty that a study tuned into the transference-countertransference dynamics in the weaning phase of a psychoanalytic psychotherapy would have definitely enriched our knowledge of the psychology of people who suffer from a pervasive developmental disorder, and would have furthered our concepts of "treatment" and "cure" applied to the psychoanalysis of such patients. In particular, I wondered whether the exit from the autistic withdrawal would correspond to a real development in their personality, or whether it were simply in a more sophisticated version of the original condition.

At this point it is possible to enhance this question, comparing two situations, with a long period of time in between. On one hand, the protocols of the five sessions which took place across the months just prior to our definitive separation, when Al was a nearly sixteen years old adolescent, and, on the other hand, the clinical observations, from when Al was a child and had received a diagnosis of autism. In the discussion I will limit myself to comparing only those aspects of the internal world of my patient that the psychoanalytic observations has made accessible to a scientific scrutiny: the symbolic processes and the relations between Infantile Self and Objects.

The "bubble" of the past and the "beliefs", the "witty remarks" and the "interests" of the present

Al arrived at his first session with me when he was just over four years old. As his mother told me in our preliminary meetings, he spent most of his time isolated from the world and from human relations, lost in a "bubble" or repetitive motor activities and idiosyncratic interests, or in an exhausting litany of self-reproaches or incomprehensible requests.

In contrast with this, he had always shown himself capable of doing jigsaw puzzles, and at certain other times he had shown reactions which seemed to contrast his autistic isolation (for example, he refused to carry on sleeping in the same room as his parents with his sister when his grandmother died and, in his place, he had brought several toys, including his favourite teddy-bear, or when he had wondered "why 'I am' crying?" whilst his mother was speaking to him on her work's office phone).

After the first few months of analysis, I had understood that his stereotypical behaviour, in which he tended to isolate himself, was the fruit of a major mastery in reproducing, precisely and delicately, several movements, gestures, people's postures and objects which had attracted his attention: of his mother (the hand movements of embroidering or adjusting the shirt collar, the manoeuvres that his mother made to park the car), of the nursery cook (the rotating movements of the wooden spoon in the polenta), the cleaning lady (cleaning the windows of the house), or of clothes hanging on the line (shaking in the wind). They were mimetic actions, which tended to be infinitely repeated.

Furthermore, I had noted that his attempts to "play" with the toys in the room were often followed by a ready-made script, and, what's more, that the game "never took off", *as if Al was unable to find in himself a "sufficient sense of conviction"*.

In the end, I had observed that following his comedown from his manic positions, either for the terror of being punished or for exhaustion, he would physically collapse, become a ragdoll or bump into the couch inappropriately. Or else, he would in contrast assume active postures, particular positions, and repeat these infinitely; he would, for example, go around the room pretending to have a limp, or stretch out on the floor pretending to be dead.

Eight years later, Al seems much changed. We discover a young adolescent who is sure of himself, anxious to do it "as a protagonist", obstinate in defending his convictions or beliefs and his interests or curiosities. Compared to the past, now he confronts and partly compares himself to other people. He is not completely closed in himself. At certain times he is capable of reflecting on his beliefs, of leaving a bit of space also for the interests and opinions of others, of measuring himself up to reality or with other points of view and with different sensitivity. Every so often, he shows that he is able to listen, correct his own errors, recognise when he doesn't know something and that he can make a mistake, accepts the reproaches and the ironies directed at him.

In brief, it could be said that whilst in the past he closed himself up in his "bubble", at this stage in his development, he seems to have acquired sufficient security in the goodness of his actions, in the intelligence of his interests and in the pleasantness of his jokes. As a result, he manages to open up the possibility of a relationship with me, using his beliefs, his interests, his jokes to surprise me, to involve me, to attract me to him, to joke with me.

From all this, one could easily jump to the conclusion that Al's current beliefs, curiosities and jokes are very different from his mimetic activities, scripts and witty remarks of the past. Unfortunately this is not completely true. Rather, even the current ones have a particular structure which remind me of his old ones: they are sequenced according to a "mathematical" logic; they seem like frames of a film or a unit of a genome, they have poor plots, subjectivity, as if they did not link in his internal world with deeper, infantile unconscious fantasies, or did not find an expansion in his imagination. I would say that they reveal all the "strength", the "energy" of subjectivity, but not the richness and individual variety, which one would expect.

The problem with his beliefs, curiosities, ironies is not therefore that of being delusional, like in the case of psychotic patients who mix up reality with fantasy, or attribute the meaning of an actual object to a symbol (the symbolic equation of A. Segal), but that they fail to find a place, a geography, a theatre (Meltzer, Harris), a room (Britton), a space in his mind to develop in complexity and quality, to be re-created by his Ego, or enriched by meanings that are shared with other Objects, internal or external. As if their music bounced or slipped off an unreceptive wall, and was continually pushed back, like an echo.

At the same time we can observe that Al, even though he is, in part, consciously using his beliefs, his scientific interests, and his witty remarks to surprise me, to put me in a good mood, to make me see that his thoughts are useful, good, lively, has a paradoxical impact on my mind and therefore on the link between our minds which is born from the fact that I am ready to share his communications. He makes me feel so "blocked" or "corked" (to use one of his terms), so exhausted, to make me lose hope that what we are doing together is useful in some way, can ever become a starting point for change. I often feel no longer able to keep up with him, and as I said before, I feel myself losing him in the mist. I am worried that he might soon disappear into his "bubble" again.

Having in mind similar situations with other patients, I would be tempted to think that he is unconsciously trying to project into me those experiences of pain and failure that belong to his infantile identity, that are very much active now in his internal world and in the transfer; that he is using me as a sort of toilet breast, with the hope that I may understand what he is going through when he feels "evil", "bad" and "stupid".

It is not like that. Why? To answer this, I have to take into account Al's reactions to my self-protective behaviour, when to survive the deadly effects of his acting out, I express to him in words and gestures, my firm decision to no longer follow him down his road. I put my foot down there and then, when for example I cover my ears so as not to listen to his impossible requests (like when he asked me whether there had been a rainy November many years ago, as there was now) or when I tease him if he insists on being entertaining, telling him that he is a "pain in the neck".

In these moments of our relationship he exhibits a strong enough "Ego" to bear the limits I impose on him, but he doesn't seem to fully grasp the motives behind my responses; he doesn't seem to be able to tune into my exhaustion, my worry, my confusion, the whole range of emotions and sensations which his behaviour brings out in me.

Instead, he feels and appreciates the strong determination, the energy, the vitality, or the lightness, the tenderness of my actions without understanding their meaning. Almost as if by magic he leaves the compartmentalised barrage of heavy fire of questions, of the absolutism of his beliefs, of the repetitiveness of his jokes. He is reanimated and gets back to work, starting to tidy up and clean his pockets and the box. He cleans the cover of the couch and sorts out my jumper so I don't "catch cold". He finally seems to be a bird that once again can fly, because it has found a bit of strength in its wings, or even a puppy, that once again can run, since it has finally shaken off the water, which was weighing down its fur.

His interest in cinematographic language and in the discovery of special effects

We can observe that Al takes inspiration for his identifications and his scripts from the world of cinematographic and television fiction. As a child, in his repetitive behaviour which would isolate him, he loved to imitate the gestures of several characters from his favourite films, like the professor Doc from *Back to the Future*; when he was older, he went further and wanted to also imitate the language of film actors, for example in his speaking in a "countrified" way, like Marisa, the character in the film *Torture Me But Fill Me up with Kisses*.

In these interests in the world of cinema, or rather, in cinematographic language, he is fascinated above all *by special effects*, by the make-up, by everything which helps to create apparitions, disappearances, transformations, leaps from one place to another, from one time to another, etc. He is interested in the tools, which allow the achievement of "magical" metamorphoses.

Furthermore, if at the start, when he was little, he wanted to "know" which materials were used to construct the special machines which were at the centre of the stories of his favourite films, like for example the time machine in *Back to the Future*, the proton pack from *Ghostbusters*, the machine to bring people back to life in *Casper*, the machine which makes children bigger and smaller in *The Little Rascals*, the machine which creates animations.

Hereafter he wants to "understand" how it is possible to record images with a recording camera and then make them visible with a projector, what has made the development from black and white films to colour films possible (colouring the frames or varying the contrast) and from silent to sound films, and therefore where the words are "stored" in dialogues that are paired with the images, what is the magic fluid which generates hypnotic states, as he saw in *Life is Beautiful* by Benigni.

His interest in the rainbow, good and bad weather, fog, artificial or natural light, the heat of light and of bodies, to which something peculiar must be added in terms of musicality: the accent of words or of phrases, not only to do with the sensorial perceptive aspects of natural phenomena, but also the tone, the crudity, the depth, the energy which they contain.

For example: indigo is not just a colour of the rainbow but it is also a tri-syllabic word, which he can play around with, stretching out the first syllable like an elastic, with a crescendo in his tone of voice which then falls into silence, *reproducing the form of a rainbow arc with his voice*. We can also observe that Al is interested in variations of intensity of the sound of the water coming out of the flush or of the sink: he can get lost in his concerts until the end of the session. I also know from material of other sessions that I have not presented here, that he likes to turn the colour of the television images on and off, using the contrast button on the remote control. He associates black and white with the degeneration of the urban suburbs in the Italian neo-realistic films, and colour with the sparkling adventures of Roger Rabbit in Toontown. Above all, he likes to surprise the cleaning lady, playing a joke of making the images on the TV disappear, whilst leaving the sound on.

It is tempting to think that the progression of these interests in cinematographic language represents the development of his "Ego": the birth of the attention and of the static memory, the recalling and the reproduction of memories, the transformation of memories with the colours and warmth of emotion, the light and the shadows, the visible and the invisible, the bridge between images and words.

Al seems interested in everything that is behind the images that he sees through his eyes or the things he perceives with his other senses, touch, smell, sounds, and makes any effort to take possession of them. But this does not mean that he is interested in understanding the meaning or in knowing the order of things. His attention is captured only by what they partake with the more elementary manifestations of life that make him feel alive, the "forms of vitality" (Stern, 2010). He seems interested in the forms of things, perceived through his senses, rather than in their emotional content.

Giving permanence and consistency to objects: writing with light

Until this point, I have tried to analyse what Al shows of himself when he tries, in his way, to impose his stunts, his jokes and his interests on me, and we have seen how difficult it is for him to leave his "script" and how every time he tries to have full control of the situation, we both run the risk of suffocating in boredom, in repetition, of slipping on the surface of his pseudoscientific beliefs.

There are, however, moments in which (see the second and third session) he is more ready to let me into his "script", to let down his "no entry" defences, to renounce his certainties and his need for perfection, to "use" his head. Then the atmosphere in the session is calm and collaborative. It is enough in this regard to observe his relationship with the calendar and with writing in general. The idea of linear time emerges with clarity and memories of past moments in his therapeutic experience emerge; the memories of a shared past becomes our story which we can meander.

In the last year of therapy, we often make references to events, behaviour, games and communications of the previous years. The feeling I get is that across the course of these years something exclusive and special for his mental life has been born inside the therapeutic process. The experience he has gone through inside the therapy room has become like a particular journey inside the more general one of his life. Any reference to this journey and its events arouses his immediate interest. Our memories are enriched by him with new details, which often help me to grasp the meaning of what I had observed many years before. At other times it is me who reminds him of something I told him in the past, which he no longer remembers. At the same time, the objects acquire *consistency and constancy* through writing in bold, or through cutting, sculpting, listening, or recording, amplifying or transcribing. It is interesting to see his writing in bold, which allow him to design the letters as though they were sculptures, a particular way of achieving a three-dimensional perspective of the object through the multiplication of the surfaces reflecting the light.

To understand the meaning of what I am saying, we must compare the three-dimensionality and the thickness of the writing and of the listening with the "*mathematical flatness*" of his predictions of how he would grow, and the "*bluntness*" of the pseudo-religious *lapidary* language with which he condemns his "sinful" mother.

The "perfection" which had a grip on his learning process, above all when he tried to understand some natural phenomena to do with things that cannot be seen, finally leaves space for their complexity (the mist, the images which are generated by electronic microchips, which come and go on the television screen, modifying the contrast). He is also continuously moving away from his "script" and more ready to try to reproduce the right conditions so he can verify certain phenomena (his shadow play on the walls which resembles the workings of a projector, his self-hypnosis), beyond a simple magical operation. He is starting to grasp that some words do not match up to real entities (ghosts, or the soul), but are the fruit of fear or of the feeling of not just being body but also "mind". He is trying to distinguish that which he manages to see with his eyes and that which is invisible (his shadow and the ghost, the fine dust against nearby light and the hypnotic flow of suggestion, the heat on the surfaces).

In these moments of calmness and sharing, the obstruction of the attention-seeking attitude, caused by his obsessive and rich catalogue or sequence of "questions", more and more often opens the door to a cloud of uncertainties and the experience of being "corked" and more rarely to a genuine wish to understand how phenomena can be reproduced.

Nonetheless, Al remains irreducibly alien to the possibility that natural phenomena, which strike a chord with him may contain an emotional significance and become the metaphor of an emotional experience (a shadow of meaning). He has just started his first steps towards the emotional experience of mirroring himself in the other, the discovery of the "otherness" in himself and the other and the possibility to imagine in his intimate relationships the first perspective of the other (what his mother feels and thinks about herself) and the third person perspective toward himself (why his mother is going to punish or forgive him).

The end of the therapy: from the isolation "in the bubble" to the indifference "of the philosopher"

All of what I have said up to this point finds a punctual confirmation in Al's actions regarding the experience of separation and of isolation, a parable which can be recapitulated in the phrase which is the title of this paragraph: *from the isolation "in the bubble" to the indifference "of the philosopher"*.

A reflection on Al's emotional orientation regarding these fundamental experiences in the development of the personality must naturally start from what his mother thinks about his apparent *indifference* towards the deaths of his grandfather and of his uncle, perhaps the most important figures in his life and who died during the last few months. She is confused and saddened by it as she was many years before, after her mother's funeral. At that time Al, who was around four, didn't seem to suffer at all for this loss in the family, and showed no need to be comforted or protected; on the contrary, instead of searching for more contact with his relatives, had suddenly changed his nocturnal habits and had refused, for the first time, to sleep with his younger sister in his parents' bedroom, where he had instead wanted to leave his toys, including his favourite teddy-bear.

Yet, again, like at the start of the therapy, the mother finds an apt description for her son's behaviour, calling him a "philosopher". She uses an expression, which seems to ring true with something in her son's deep, emotional life, which had happened before; when describing his social and personal isolation, she called him "the boy in the bubble". I say "seems", because, across the years, I learned that the "bubble" had its own structure; it was quite a complicated metaphor that did not simply mean that something was lacking. In this way I also suspect that the image of the "philosopher's" indifference may have a deeper substance than one might first think.

All of us, including his mother, are used to thinking that the loss of a dear person or thing is a painful experience, as we can easily observe in small children who burst into tears when they can no longer see their mother or when they meet a stranger or think that they have lost their favourite toy. We are expecting to glean the same suffering in those who are grieving. This all seems very obvious, which is why we worry so much when, in a similar situation, we observe a lack of a sorrowful emotional reaction. The indifference is immediately perceived as something unnatural, something we cannot easily understand, a sort of insult to something fundamental in human relationships. After all, we know that even elephants cry and watch over the dead members of their group. *We have a mixed reaction of fear, disapproval and blame towards this indifference.*

However, as Freud has shown in Appendix C of *Inhibitions, Symptoms and Anxiety* (1926d [1925]), speaking of the main emotional reactions to a loss of an object, the psychology of these emotional processes is anything but simple to describe. He writes that there are still many questions in this area of human experience, which demand an answer: "Why are loss and grief so painful? How can we put the painful reaction, which accompanies this experience, into perspective? What happens in the human mind when the separation or the loss of a loved one or an interesting object generates anguish, or perhaps only grief and even, only sadness"—and, I would add—indifference?

Freud, in the above article, links loss and grief to the ability of the subject to develop a praiseworthy, passionate, emotional investment in the object, over and above the purely narcissistic interests which would bring alone, at the moment of loss and the mourning, the emotional experience of a "insatiable and nostalgic longing" to have it still and forever.

In this regard, Melanie Klein wrote about depressive pain, connecting it to the depressive position, a developmental phase of the emotionality in the first year of life, characterised by the "pining for the lost loved object" (Klein, 1935, 1940), differentiating this painful emotional experience from other types of anguish and pathological depression, linked to the paranoid-schizoid position.

In which way can we use these psychoanalytical concepts and observations to explain Al's "indifference"? Should we think that it has something to do with his failure to reach the depressive position? Or should these interpretations give way to different developmental scenarios?

At this point I think it is important to summarise what emerges from the clinical material in the last year of therapy, respecting the chronology of events.

First of all, we can observe the way in which Al tries to give a personal meaning to the two changes in the therapeutic context: the loss of the second weekly session and the end of the therapy. He links it to his way of looking at life in general terms, which comes up quite clearly, in his reply to a direct question of mine on this topic: he tells me that for him life is just a quiz where you win or you lose by pure luck.

A few months later, he turns to the same life philosophy to tell me that I had been "lucky" that his mother had decided to take away the promised punishment of not taking him to the seaside anymore, which had made him feel furious. He does not seem capable of understanding that my suggestions arose from my knowledge of how the "heart" of his "sinful" mother would work, and at the same time, of admitting his own fault. His mother's severity seems to him incomprehensible and unpredictable, like "the lightning strike" from the scene with "Doc": one can only be frightened of it.

The theme of the goodbye' appears again in his reflections in the film *Torture Me, But Fill Me up with Kisses*, directed by the Italian Dino Risi in 1968. To speak the truth, the film contains two goodbyes, one romantic and agonising, and the other full of hatred and resentment, which both belong to, Marino and Marisa, the two main protagonists of the film, which go from the position of heroic lovers, both fighting against anyone who stands in the way of their passion, to those of disappointed lovers who have to face the prospect of betrayal (on his part). Al mostly likes to imitate Marisa's "countrified" language in this script, transferring it to the phrase "I don't give a toss about Dr B", to communicate amusingly and wittily *how aware he is that the therapy is ending*.

His awareness of the end of the therapy and of time passing towards the last session, is always present in recent months in the calendar game, and also in his concentration, which he dedicates first to highlighting and then to crossing out the date which corresponds to the day of the session. In addition to all this, we can observe a moment in which the idea of the end of the therapy becomes a source of worry, when he asks me if without the therapy he will ever be able to manage his "bad behaviour", identifying a regulating and protective function in the therapy which, he fears, he could eventually miss after its end.

However, this awareness is not coupled with a profound affective commonality. Towards the world of the mind, that is, the emotional experience of dependence and separation belonging to internal and external object relationships, Al seems to have the same ritualistic, factual information based and detached attitude that children show in their religious feelings towards the supernatural.

I am particularly referring to research conducted by Castiglioni in the first half of the twentieth century, the subject of God among children (1928) and on the religious feelings of adolescents (1949), which bring two very different certainties under discussion. The first one being that great natural phenomena determine a particular state of harmony with divinity in a child's psyche, and the second one that states that the experienced feelings of the child in their religious experiences is completely similar to that of an adult.

Castiglioni maintains, on the other hand, that there is no evidence that children spontaneously associate the perception of natural, particularly violent phenomena (such as lightning), to a supernatural entity. At the same time, he asserts that if a supernatural world exists for a child, this is an independent world in itself because, although it is present in the child's awareness, it does not affect him; it is not subject to his actions.

R. Vianello (1980 [1991]) carried out research into the principal characteristics of children's religiousness in the eras of preschool, school, and the early years of adolescence (and on representations of divinity, beliefs in a Creator, in a God which guarantees justice and immortality). He concludes in his results that fantasies about relations between the everyday world and God's supernatural world are conditioned (and, in turn, they slow down evolution) by several fundamental tendencies of children's brains such as realism, magic, animism, as they were described by Jean Piaget in numerous books published between 1923 and 1932.

He shows how the totality of notions, which children learn through religious instruction, are assimilated in a disorganised and incoherent way based on factual knowledge and, in addition, they often clash with beliefs stemming from everyday life. "In other terms", he writes (Vianello, 1980, p. 63), "the information available to us suggest that *a child's religious experience is neither essential nor dynamic (or only in a very small part), because it does not invest sufficiently the children affectivity (or it fails to do so homogeneously enough) so to compose (or restructure) a personality in a way which matches up to religious beliefs* [italics in the original text]. A child's experiences (of the sacred and terrestrial), therefore, seem to belong to two different levels of reality, which little contact between them."

In light of these digressions, we can perhaps better understand why Al does not associate the perception of a few natural phenomena with his personal emotions, and why he is apparently indifferent towards death and separation, proving that he acts towards the world of the mind in the same ritualistic and slightly adhesive way in which children act towards the supernatural.

The bridge towards the immaterial

At this point we might ask ourselves: is there any evidence, in the clinical material, that in the course of these years therapy has modified, at least in part, the lack of imaginative space in Al's internal world?

Up to this point, our discussion might suggest a negative answer. However, it is important to see how in the final period of therapy Al was able to get access to the world of emotions, how he managed to grasp the concept of linear time and some notion of depth and perspective, and how he was able to discover some shared meanings.

My hypothesis is that he was able to reach such important objectives for his mental and psychic life by following a pathway that is quite different from ours, by means of different modalities of research and conceptual instruments, which allowed him to achieve them, nevertheless; and the final result of his development, despite its being a way of existing in this world that is ill-suited to the intimate dimension of human relationships, must be understood and respected. My impression is that the mother's (or carer's) failure to acknowledge or to accept this particular pathway from the earliest stages of the neonatal life of a baby suffering from pervasive developmental disorder, may lead to the introjection of a Superego that is very sadistic in its demand for perfection and adaptation.

I seem to be able to confirm that in all these years of therapy, my relationship with Al has advanced on two levels: on one hand, that of reducing the destructivity of the "perfection" of the Superego, and on the other hand, that of reawakening his emotional life. However, whilst I am aware of the interpretative function, which I exercised in reducing both the sadistic and delusional aspects of the supposed perfection of his Superego, and also the omnipotent part of his infantile Self, and the benefits that are derived from stabilising his mood, experiencing serenity, giving new strength to his epistemophilic instinct. It has been much more difficult to understand how successful it has been to help him to access a normal and emotional life (firstly to my normal and emotional life), and above all to appreciate it and to make it a source of his mental life, a stimulus to his imagination.

I intuitively think, however, that the two functions are linked.

A suggestive synthesis can be found in the modality with which Al reacts to separation, to loss and to grief at the very end of his therapy. We see how he, at a certain point in the penultimate session when talking about the writing ATR, reacts when I tell him that "A" (for Al) has spent many years with his therapist "R" (for Roberto) trying to understand the difference between using his head "T", (from "testa" in Italian, head) to think his own thoughts and emotions and, on the contrary, to act out his own fears and rages, closing himself in the bubble of perfection of magic and pseudoscientific and religious simplifications. That our work together has mostly consisted of learning how to protect his own relations, the most important ones being with his parents and teachers, against the impulse of immediately putting up "no entry" signs as soon as he felt confronted with the inadequacy of his own knowledge and with the "infernal" scolding for his punishments.

I will add that we have managed to successfully differentiate his mental states and several characters, which he likes to interpret, but we have only partially shared their emotional meaning. We can observe in these moments an acceleration in his development, an intensification of the introjective processes which are the foundation of the world of recollections and memory. He is very interested in light which makes things visible with the eyes and perceptible to touch, in shadows or in fog, which, in contrast to the light, generates a mysterious world of ghosts and of the soul, in colours, which, like particular rays of light, in contrast with the black and white, as Vittorio Storaro (2010) says, have a soul: the azure of the sea (which is also the colour of my eyes), the blue of the felt-tip (the colour of magic and power), orange, the complexion of Jessica Rabbit (the colour of passion and sensuality), the grey of fog (the colour of waiting, of the suspension of life), the black of Neorealism in Italian black-and-white cinema (the colour of suburbs, of abandonment and disrepair).

At the same time he is interested in voices, in sounds, in tones, in noises, as if he were starting to appreciate the importance of listening, in which he seems busy treating what is said, recording it, transcribing it, amplifying it, not letting it disperse, disappear into nothing; he wants to offer it the support of images because they live longer. *Al continues to write his life primarily with light and with material, and still seldom with feelings and emotions.*

The poem by Tagore from the collection *Fruit Gathering*, quoted at the beginning of this book, has a second verse which contains, in my opinion, a profound idea of what are the path towards true knowledge and the creative act: both of them are like the "blooming of a bud and its becoming a flower". This is a wonderful image of what a transformation is, a metaphor of an awakening to life in the encounter with God in religion, and of the birth of the mind in the therapeutic relationship.

It is used by Tagore also in other lyrics, always filling it with new meanings.

In this poem the great Indian poet seems to warn "he who cannot": one cannot make a flower bloom by simply touching, jerking or shaking it. One needs to wait for the heat of the morning, the summer sun, the bliss of light, the breath of all things to set the bud free. Thus, we therapists must also be able to patiently wait for the beauty of the world and the internal objects to free the fragile infantile Self of the children and adolescents who suffer from pervasive developmental disorders and lead it towards life.

> [...] He who can open the bud does it so simply.
> He gives it a glance,
> and the life-sap stirs through its veins.
> At his breath the flower spreads its wings and flutters in the wind.
> Colours flush out like heart-longings, the perfume betrays a sweet secret.
> He who can open the bud does it so simply. (Tagore, 1916, p. XVIII)

APPENDICES A TO K

Areas of conceptual and methodological development

In the following section I will try to offer a clearer definition of the conceptual tools, which I applied to the clinical notes in the book while interpreting the behaviour of my patients. In doing so I hope to help people who are not familiar with the observational method of child psychoanalysis to share my way of looking at the developing mind in children and at the same time to allow those colleagues or other professionals who are already accustomed to it to test its usefulness in future research and therapeutic work.

Appendix A: the alpha-function

The alpha-function is a fundamental concept in W. R. Bion's "theory of thinking", according to which, in order to "learn from experience", the individual must transform the sense impressions of early emotional experiences (beta elements) into psychic elements (alpha elements). The notion of alpha-function was first introduced in *Learning from Experience* (1962) on the notion that any knowledge of the human mind, even the most abstract one, is largely metaphorical, and that the earliest metaphors used are those that can date back to sensorial experience and to the perceptions of our sensory-motor apparatus. In this sense, any theory on the birth and development of the mind must be seen as a hypothesis, whose validity lies in its capacity to enhance the quality of our observations of clinical phenomena; therefore it has the significance of a model that, when no longer useful to its purpose, must be abandoned.

In the third chapter on "The eyes and the mind" I have made a few examples of this transformative process (the working of the alpha-function) that W. R. Bion talks about, in the encounter between the mind of a photographer-artist and the natural environment around him, in the music and dance that sustains the encounter of the eyes of a mother and the movements of her "little rascal", in Tagore's poems on the birth and death of a child, and in the interpretative activity of a therapist who tries to give meaning to his own personal experiences, which are linked to the conscious and unconscious communications of his little patient Richard. In the book there is another reference to the working of alpha-function and its main factors, in the discussion of the dream of the three elephants (in the clinical case of Rebecca.), in which dreaming is seen as a process leading towards the discovery of the meaning of emotional experiences, particularly of those linked to the beauty and truth of early object relations.

Appendix B: the notion of reverie

The term reverie, which is used to frame our ideas on the birth and growth of the mind, reverberates with several meanings. I use it to highlight a particular quality of the adult—mainly maternal—attitude in apprehending what in intersubjective communication belongs to projective identification, regardless of the instruments with which it manifests itself and the contents that it carries. The most interesting example of this is that of the mother of the "little rascal", where some of the child's physical behaviours become the expression of a lively intentionality.

Reverie is a mode of listening, ample and open, concerning the most primitive physical states of which a child can be aware; it manifests itself through all the senses of the person who experiences it: sight, hearing, touch, and movement. It is an amplifying, receptive, predisposition, which, in the discovery of psychic reality, performs the same function as the large astronomical telescopes in the exploration of sidereal space, which is apparently static, empty and silent. It helps one's eyes to see further, to reach something that goes beyond appearances; it supports the "awareness" that the Other has of himself or herself in a state of general empathic identification.

A very plastic conjecture on the function of the reverie of the maternal mind was described by Money-Kyrle in a post-scriptum (1977) to "Cognitive Development" (1968): through the interpretation of a dream, the author shows how a mother's capacity for reverie—and similarly of a therapist in the transference—may help a child (or a patient alike), in his growth, to develop a capacity to overcome some of the most primitive obstacles in his normal cognitive development.

Appendix C: the notion of reversal of the alpha-function

From a mathematical viewpoint, a function can be seen as an input-output device, i.e., something that takes an object as input and produces another as output. This happens according to a very precise, univocal prescription, so that the same input leads to the same output. However, the opposite does not happen. Usually the function works only in one direction—the arrow that goes from left to right defines the function—from the output one cannot go back to the input.

How can we, then, use the notion of alpha function working in reverse in the framework of psychological clinical phenomena? What sense does it make to talk about inversion, of change of direction? The answer can be formulated thus: instead of transforming beta into alpha elements and use them to build the contact barrier of alpha elements which is crucial for the differentiation between the internal and the external world, the alpha-function working in reverse attacks and disperses the contact barrier (the matrix of thinking), creating objects that are quite different from the original beta elements that Bion calls bizarre objects (1957). Such objects contain "traces of the Ego and the Superego": i.e., they have the "complexion" of the personality they originate from.

In *Explorations in Autism*, Meltzer (1975a, p. 217) envisages the possibility that some emotional experiences dismantled by primitive obsessional mechanisms of an autistic kind to a level of simplicity below common sense, may no longer function as "symbolic forms" containing emotional meaning, and may in fact resemble—in their most *extreme instances*—Bion's "bizarre objects". A clinical example of this is presented in Chapter Three, when I describe the script with which my patient Al attempts to convert me to his belief in the transmigration of the soul; from this illustration, one can see how the interests, objects, and viewpoints on internal and external reality of patients like him are all affected by "restrictions and constraints", and how the capacity for reverie of their internal and external objects is altered and replaced by a kind of attention that oscillates between two anti-developmental polarities, between lack of attention and automatic mimicry. These notions can be analysed in more depth in Chapter Five, where I quoted several excerpts from Caccia's paper (2012) on the "Distinction between primitive and psychotic in early object relations", in which it is clear how important it is, in the study of the development and psychopathology of mental life, to recognise the difference between what has never become unconscious from what has become so, as well as what has been dreamt first, and then turned into a bizarre object.

Appendix D: the clinical phenomenon of negative contagion

The term negative contagion is introduced in the book to indicate a peculiar aspect of the countertransference in psychoanalytic work with children and adolescents suffering from pervasive developmental disorders that becomes visible when the personality of the therapist clashes with the two-dimensional functioning of the patients. I have assigned to it a syndromic meaning underlying a possible correspondence with a cataplexy, a somatic and neurological phenomenon. When negative contagion occurs, the therapist finds himself into a mind—his own—that is completely devoid of images to hold on to; he feels like falling, suddenly and relentlessly, into a state of mental death which is foreign to him but that appear to be justified by the events in which he is actively participating in the relationship with his patient.

We have seen that the main defences of the therapist against the experience of feeling hurt, incapable, and disabled in his capacity to image what is going on inside the analytic experience, are the automatic recording of events and interpretative solipsism. We can observe how in the first case the process of knowing the Other, which is the basis for any human link—and therefore also the analytic one—is completely dominated by an objective viewpoint (the patient as an object of study), while in the second case it is replaced by a "view" of the facts which is altogether subjective, and almost arbitrary. What is remarkably missing in either case is the aesthetic viewpoint; in the relationship the experience of aesthetic reciprocity is not activated (see Chapter Nine).

As a way to get an understanding of the phenomenon of negative contagion, I would like to suggest to read what in his book, *Lo Sguardo del Flaneur* (2002), Ulf Peter Hallberg, a modern Swedish writer, wrote about his visit to the exhibition *The White Room. The Void* by the French artist Yves Klein, a representative of the post-modern artistic school called "nouveau realisme", very well known for his monochrome painting.

Hallberg writes:

> The room is about four metres wide and three metres high [...]. Two neon lamps are hanging from the ceiling. Walls and ceiling are covered with white paint; everything is blindingly white [...] when the white lock closes behind you, nothing can help you anymore. You feel out of this world, in an intermediate realm, more alone than one could possibly imagine. You cannot rely on anything, not even the four solid walls around you: they fade into a white fog, in a brightness that conveys a sense of infinity ... you are in the middle of all this, lost, and you try to come back to your senses: a human being destined to die. (Hallberg, 2002, p. 46)

The white room is an art object that annihilates the dimension of space, projecting the Ego into the only remaining dimension: that of an infinite time, which—when one "wakes up"—conveys an intolerably painful awareness of one's finiteness, solitude, and death.

Appendix E: the notion of part object

The notion of part object was born and developed within the theory of object relations in the British school of psychoanalysis, and it is fundamentally important both in the establishment of a psychoanalytic theory of normal emotional and mental development and in the understanding of more serious and debilitating psychopathological clinical manifestations. It is an integral part of a wider set of concepts that try to delineate a particular aspect of the mental functioning of an individual, a group or an institution, which Melanie Klein called paranoid-schizoid position, that specifically contributes to the general processes of learning from experience and of reality testing. The first object relation that a baby establishes with his mother is not with a whole object, but with parts of it; similarly, the experience that the baby has of himself, his body and its contents, is partial. From the very beginning of life, these fragmented and partial experiences are influenced by some very primitive mental processes, erroneously called defence mechanisms, such as splitting, idealisation, projection, introjection, and projective identification, through which the Ego of the child tries to give some order to the chaos and fragmentation of his experience, resorting to the help of his mother in this arduous task.

Appendix F: compositional aspects of communication

In my psychoanalytical work with very disturbed adolescents, borderline and borderline-psychotic (Bertolini, 1998) I have realised that in order to revive my patients' hope to "be understood", and their capacity to accept the truth of what is given back to them of what they have express of themselves, it was necessary to introduce some specific compositional elements in the attention, the general attitude and the interpretative comments of the therapist, like the right distance, the right speed, the right temperature, the right weight, the right consistency, the right rhythm ... which are so important in painting, music, and dance. For example, in Chapter Eight, I showed how Rebecca's deep link with the nipple/breast, as a part object, within the analytic relationship, was hindered by a twofold negative experience: on one hand that of a hard nipple, experienced as penetrating and hurtful, and on the other that of a soft, inconsistent nipple that could not be grasped.

In my 1998 paper, I pointed out how these compositional aspects can be studied by analysing the behaviours of mothers and fathers when they look after their children, relate to them when they are distressed, communicate with them when they are happy and try to interpret their behaviours in their early months of life. Observing the parents not in what they do, but in the way they "get round" the needs and wishes of their children, when they attach them to the breast, comfort them, protect them, dress them, clean them and put them to bed, one will find something that regulates and modulates such activities; a mental state that accompanies them, a sort of mental quality: a common denominator that I have called the compositional aspect of intersubjective communication.

In more disturbed patients, one has the feeling that something essential has been missed in the compositional aspects of their intersubjective human experience in their first months of life, in the way their objects tried to "read" and make "legible" their way of being; somehow, therefore, their relationship with themselves, particularly with their body and with reality, suffered, from the very start, from "restrictions and constrictions". In extreme cases, this led to the inability to communicate externally and to dream in the internal world. To this regard, it might be interesting to investigate, as I have already done in Chapter Eight, the dream about the elephants, not from an iconographic perspective but from the viewpoint of its compositional elements, in order to try to consider more clearly the features of the tail and the trunk in a three-dimensional and four-dimensional perspective, just as we might look at Munch's *Scream*, and discover that what we see in the foreground—the face and the gesture of the hands on the ears of the character—take on a symbolic, universal meaning because of the way in which they are part of a landscape, arranged in a scene, because of the distances between the various narrative planes, and the chromatic effect of the colours. Thus, looking at the painting, one immediately feels the power of unheeded suffering.

How can a painting speak? How can its iconographic aspect evoke in us such intense emotions and make us hear a silent scream? How can it make us get closer to the unheeded suffering of the character in the foreground to the point that it gives meaning to his painful experience, a meaning that also belongs to our everyday life, or to the atmosphere that characterises the social links of a whole generation? We truly discover how art helps us retrieve an emotional experience through the artist's internal work and its external disclosure in the painting.

Appendix G: the concepts of misconception and disorientation in object relations

The theory of misconceptions and disorientations can be found in Roger Money-Kyrle's "Cognitive development" (1968), one of his most inspired papers. Here, the author describes the difficulties experienced by some of his patients in psychic reality—and consequently in the analytic transference—in orientating the most primitive aspects of their personality towards a loved object, in identifying themselves with it both at a part-object level—the breast-nipple—or as a whole: the mother, or the relationship, not only of a sexual nature, between the parents. His assumption is that the baby, just like all the other animals, is naturally predisposed to find out the truth about the facts of life, and that for this reason he is equipped from birth with the ability to find his bearings and recognise his own objects of dependence—at first the good breast-nipple, and then the good relationship, not only sexual, of his parents. Money-Kyrle rejects the idea that at birth the mind of the baby is a *tabula rasa*; instead, just like Bion, he thinks that it is provided with innate preconceptions of good objects of dependence. He associates this innate preconception to something that exists but cannot be imagined: an "empty thought" that is shaped or filled by the encounter with an object in real life, through the experience of recognition. It is as if in the encounter with the breast of the mother, the child thought: "I have found what I was looking for", just like we finally retrieve a lost word in our memory. Starting from these assumptions, R. M. Kyrle wonders about what might prevent, in the encounter between the mind of the child and reality, the transformation of the innate preconception of a good object into its conception, which has something to do with the "thought of", the "memory of" it. He notices that (such notions appear in a person's development) with different levels of representation (concrete, ideographic and verbal) and awareness, and that if innate preconceptions do not find a realisation, they may, in certain situations, leave room for misconceptions, distortions.

According to the author, the obstacles to the supremacy of the reality and truth of experience—to the acknowledgement of which the child is naturally predisposed—are mainly of an emotional nature, linked to the child's own temperament, or to birth-related traumatic facts, or to aspects of emotional and sensorial deprivation in the baby's early periods of post-natal life. In addition to all this, R. M. Kyrle claims that the child, passionately caught by these realisations, will try to place his good dependence objects in a space-time system, a geography which will initially belong to his external world and then, as the consequence of the latter's internalisation, to his internal world. In normal development, the good breast-nipple will become the basis of the child's attention, the centre of his mental geography, around which the first space-time divisions will develop: the period of realisation (being fed); the period of remembering (having been fed); and the period of waiting (going to be fed). In pathological personalities, the orientation towards a good basis can easily be lost, both at an internal and an external level, in various ways that will manifest themselves in different forms of disorientation and confusion.

Making reference to these concepts was important in the study of my patients' infantile transference, since it helped me keep alive the idea that the autistic part of a pervasive disorder should not be considered *tout court* as an absence, but as a deficit in the conception of the Other, the consequence of a space-time disorientation in the geography of the mind which prevents these patients from getting access to an intimate relationship with another human being, at least in the way we are used to considering it.

Appendix H: the concept of claustrum

Generally, the term claustrum evokes the image of an enclosed, silent place, where one can walk, meditate, and pray: a place that, like the consultation room, helps individuals to get deeply in touch with themselves and their internal objects.

Meltzer (1992) however, uses the term claustrum to describe a place that is no longer part of life and is confused with the ill mind of the people who inhabit it.

In this book, I apply the term claustrum to some specific configurations of infantile transference within the analytic relationship of my very disturbed children or adolescent patients (see the clinical material of S and Re), when they live in the therapy room as if it were the inside of the body/mind of the mother and confound me, or parts of me, with very persecutory or eroticised objects, like the nipple-penis in the breast, or the penis-baby in mother's genitals/bottom. In such situations, the boundary or the difference between Self and object is completely erased, and the awareness of the differences between psychic reality and external reality is obliterated for more or less lengthy periods.

Appendix I: the concepts of intransigent and faulty objects

I was able to describe in my book how the interests of my patients were hindered by "constrictions and restrictions", dominated as they were by an outlook on reality which was too idiosyncratic and at same time too superficial. In the clinical case of Alessio, I have illustrated the importance of these concepts, when I analysed the request for perfection (which has to do with constriction) and for simplification (which has to do with restriction), that originated from his internal and external objects of dependence, or from the child's infantile Self, often confused with them, which dominated his conception of intimate relationships and of the causal links of physical reality, and which prevented him from participating, more directly and personally, in a deep human link, and from making science in an original manner.

Appendix J: significant form and aesthetic emotion

In various parts of this book I have highlighted the importance of investigating the processes that underlie the symbolic representation of reality—particularly artistic reality—and of studying those that guide human creativity. In my prologue I have stated that the most painful discovery in my first encounters with children suffering from disorders of the autistic spectrum was the realisation that what in the animal kingdom usually creates proximity, interest, intimacy, and performs a function of calling and courtship, i.e., beauty, harmony of movement, order, colour, and song, remains extraneous to any communicative and social intentionality, imprisoned in an unfathomable solipsism, unable to arouse any aesthetic emotion. This has led me to elaborate what some authors have written on aesthetic experiences linked to visual arts, and to think that there may be something in the behaviour of my patients which does not take a shape that might somehow stimulate such experiences in them.

In this sense, I found Clive Bell's notion of *significant form* quite useful, when applied to the birth and evolution of the early artistic expressions. The notion of "significant form" was first used by Clive Bell (1881–1964) in a small book entitled *Art* (1914), to define the quality shared by all the works of art—particularly the visual arts—that can arouse an aesthetic emotion in us because of their "beauty". In *The Path of Beauty: A Study of Chinese* Li Zehou (1988) talks about beauty as a significant form, a natural form that has acquired, in time, a socially definite content and has become the representation of subjective feelings.

I could then claim that my patients have an awareness of reality that is irrespective (in different degrees, from case to case) of its symbolic representation as a "significant form".

I must confess that for a long time, being neither an artist nor a historian of visual arts, I have struggled to appreciate these notions and to utilise them in order to conceptualise my clinical experience, particularly in the study of the evolution of the transference and the countertransference. There was, however, a recent experience that helped me comprehend them better. During a long walk in the Libyan region of the Tadrad Acacus, an area that had been inhabited by man before becoming a desert, I left my group of fellow travellers to spend some time in complete solitude, when I suddenly noticed a stone whose shape was different from all the ones I had seen until then. I got closer and I picked it up. As I looked at it from very close, I immediately realised that it was a piece of wrought flint, an artefact (my guide later told me that it was probably an object used for skinning animals). I experienced a great emotion as I noticed that it perfectly fitted my hand and its movements. I felt that something had bridged the gap between whoever had made it and me, conveying a deep feeling of shared identity.

Realising that such a stone was an artefact because of its shape, and also because of the functions that it mobilised in my Ego when I held it in my hand, made me experience a particular emotion, which I will never forget, that I can only define as aesthetic: what I felt through my senses in that moment, immediately put me in touch with the "mind" of my forefather who had carved it.

I became aware that aesthetic emotion does not only belong to the apprehension of the beauty of a work of art, but also to the form and the function of human artefacts (consider the importance of beauty in the design of Apple computers); also, if I think back to my experience as a secondary school student, I remember how, alongside the beauty of a poem, I also was able to discover the beauty of a mathematical formula, or of a geometric theorem. For this reason, in my book I have tried to describe both viewpoints about my patients: that of the construction of psychic reality and that of the transformation of external reality.

Appendix K: perspective as a symbolic "form"

In "Dimensionality as a parameter of mental functioning; its relation to narcissistic organization", D. Meltzer (1975b) wrote that a living organism can have a mental life only if it manages to have a notion of "space" as a "life space" (Kurt Lewin), not as a void, but as a whole that is inseparable from the characters and the objects that inhabit it. A place (space) where events (time) and emotionally relevant encounters occur, which become the metaphors of a link, and where one can meet people and objects that, because of their form and nature, lend themselves to becoming transference objects. As I wrote this book, in several moments, I realised how important it was to observe the ways the patients perceive and envisage the space and the events in which they are immersed within the consultation room and try to communicate something about themselves through their movements, posture and gaze.

Particularly in the clinical cases of S the little Goldilocks, and of Re, the child kissed by the Snow Queen, we have been able to follow the path of development of the infantile transference which allowed them to get out of a two-dimensional mental condition and to get access to an experience of space as a life-space, and of time as linear time.

Their gaze on the Object and the gaze of the Object on them became "a congruent construction of a relational model" (Gombrich), or an act of "Soul-making" (Keats) through the conquest of a three-dimensional notion of the Object itself (R's sculptures) and the relinquishment of special perspectives (linked to obsessional mechanisms of a primitive kind, like the dismantling and reversal of the alpha function—see Chapter Four).

What I found important for the conceptualisation of these internal movements was the reading of the studies of Erwin Panofsky (1927) on "perspective as a symbolic form" and of the psycho-perceptive research on the nature of the space of the psychology of form by R. Arnheim (1954) and E. H. Gombrich (1996) and of the books of Meg Harris Williams, mainly the most recent one on *The Aesthetic Development* (2010b).

REFERENCES

Alvarez, A. (1992). *Live Company: Psychoanalytic Psychotherapy with Autistic, Borderline, Deprived and Abused Children*. London: Routledge.

Alvarez, A. (2004). Finding the Wavelength. Tools in communication with children with Autism. *The International Journal of Infant Observation and its Applications, volume 7, nos. 2 & 3*: 91–106. London: The Tavistock Clinic Foundation in association with Lawrence and Wishart Ltd.

Alvarez, A. (2012). *The Thinking Heart: Three Levels of Psychoanalytic Therapy with Disturbed Children*, London: Routledge.

Alvarez, A., & Reid, S. (Eds.) (1999). *Autism and Personality: Findings from the Tavistock Autism Workshop*. London: Routledge.

Arnheim, R. (1954). *Art and Visual Perception—a Psychology of the Creative Eye*. Berkeley Los Angeles: California University.

Arshavsky, Y. I. (2003). Cellular and network properties in the functioning of the nervous system: from central pattern generators to cognition. *Brain Research Review, 41*: 229–267.

Associazione Culturale Racker Venezia (2002). *Considerazioni attuali sull'Autismo*. Gruppo di studio e approfondimento della teoria delle relazioni oggettuali in psicoanalisi. Typescript, 23rd November 2002, p. 3. Translated for this edition by Aldo Grassi: Oxford.

Bell, C. (1914). *Art*. London: Chatto & Windus.

Bergson, H. L. (1919). *L'Énergie spirituelle, Essais et Conferences,* Paris, Librairie Felix Alcan. H. Wildon Carr (Trans.). *Mind-energy, a Collection of Essays and Lectures*. London: McMillan and Company, 1920.

Bertolini, R. (1998). The light meter, the thermostat, the tuner: the compositional aspects of communication with very disturbed adolescents. In: M. Cohen & A. Hahn (Eds). *Exploring the work of Donald Meltzer* (pp. 103–118). London: Karnac, 2000.

Bick, E. (1964). Notes on infant observation in psycho-analytic training. *International Journal of Psychoanalysis, 45*: 558–566.

Bion, W. R. (1948). *Experiences in groups, Human Relations, vols. I–IV, 1948–1951*. Reprinted in *Experiences in Groups* (1961). London: Tavistock.

Bion, W. R. (1950). The imaginary twin. *Second Thoughts*. London: Heinemann.

Bion, W. R. (1955). The development of schizophrenic thought. *International Journal of Psychoanalysis, 37*, also in *Second Thoughts* (1967).

Bion, W. R. (1957). The differentiation of the psychotic from the non-psychotic personalities. *International Journal of Psychoanalysis, 38*, also in *Second Thoughts* (1967).

Bion, W. R. (1959). Attacks on linking. *International Journal of Psychoanalysis, 40*(5–6). Also in: *Second Thoughts* (1967).

Bion, W. R. (1962). *Learning from Experience*. London: William Heinemann.

Bion, W. R. (1963). *The Elements of Psycho-Analysis*. London: Heinemann (1963); Karnac (1984).

Bion, W. R. (1967). *Second Thoughts*. London: Heinemann (1967); Karnac (1984).

Bion, W. R. (1970). Container and contained transformed. *Attention and Interpretation*. London: Tavistock Publications Limited.

Bion, W. R. (1982). *The Long Weekend 1897–1919: Part of a Life*. London: Karnac.

Bion, W. R. (1983). *Bion in Rome (Seminari Italiani)*. Rome: Borla, 1985, p. 14. Translated for this edition by Aldo Grassi: Oxford.

Bion, W. R. (1992). *Cogitations*. F. Bion (Ed.). London: Karnac.

Bobath, B. (1965). *Abnormal Postural Reflex Activity Caused by Brain Lesions*. London: Heinemann.

Bodei, R. (2008). *Paesaggi sublimi*. Milano: Bompiani. Translated for this edition by Aldo Grassi: Oxford.

Britton, R. (1999). *Belief and Imagination: Explorations in Psychoanalysis*. London: Routledge.

Caccia, O. (2012). Differenze fra primitivo e psicotico nello sviluppo mentale del bambino. *Richard & Piggle, 2012, vol. 1*. Il pensiero Scientifico, pp. 66–85. Translated for this edition by Aldo Grassi: Oxford.

Castiglioni, G. (1945). *Il ritorno della Psicologia*. Brescia: *Scuola e Vita*. Translated for this edition by Aldo Grassi: Oxford.

Clark, P. (1933). *The Nature and Treatment of Amentia*. New York: Bailliere.

Freud, S. (1895d). *Studies on Hysteria. SE, 2*. London: Hogarth Press.

Freud, S. (1917). Mourning and Melancholia. *SE, 14*. London: Hogarth Press.

Freud, S. (1923b). *The Ego and the Id. SE, 19*. London: Hogarth Press.

Freud, S. (1926d [1925]). *Inhibitions, Symptoms and Anxiety. SE, 20*. London: Hogarth Press.

Gombrich, E. H. (1996). *The Essential Gombrich. Selected Writings on Art and Culture*. London: Phaidon Press Limited.

Hallberg, U. P. (2002). *Lo sguardo del Flaneur*. [Original title: Flanoerens Blick, Norstedts Foerlag, Stockholm, 1966]. Milano: Iperborea, p. 46. Translated for this edition by Aldo Grassi: Oxford.

Harris, M. (1977). *The Tavistock Training and Philosophy, Collected Papers of M. Harris and E. Bick*. The Roland Harris Educational Trust, 1987.

Harris, P. L. (1989). Children and Emotion. The development of Psychological Understanding, Chapter 9, In: *Autism*, pp. 193–215. Oxford: Blackwell Publisher.

Houzel, D. (2004). The psychoanalysis of infantile autism. *Journal of Child Psychotherapy, 30*(2): 225–237.

Hoxter, S. (1975). The Residual Autistic Condition and its Effect upon Learning. *Explorations in Autism, a Psychoanalytical Study*. The Roland Harris Educational Trust. Perthshire: Clunie Press.

Joseph, B. (1989). *Psychic Equilibrium and Psychic Change*. London: Routledge.

Keats, J. (1970). *Selected Letters*. R.Gittings (Ed.). Oxford: Oxford University Press.

Klein, M. (1927). Symposium on child-analysis. *International Journal of Psychoanalysis, 8*: 339–370.

Klein, M. (1931). A contribution to the theory of intellectual inhibition. *International Journal of Psychoanalysis, 12*: 206–218.

Klein, M. (1935). A contribution to the psychogenesis of manic-depressive states. *International Journal of Psychoanalysis, 16*: 145–174.

Klein, M. (1940). Mourning and its relation to manic-depressive states. *International Journal of Psychoanalysis, 21*: 125–153.

Klein, M. (1946). Notes on Some Schizoid Mechanisms. *International Journal of Psychoanalysis, 27*: 99–110.

Maiello Hunziker, S. (1986). *Esperienze di psicoterapia infantile: il modello Tavistock*. Firenze: Martinelli, p. 80. Translated for this edition by Aldo Grassi: Oxford.

Mancia, M. (1981). On the beginning of mental life in the foetus. *International Journal of Psychoanalysis, 62*: 351–357.

Mannoni, M. (1964). *L'enfant arriéré et sa mère. Paris. The Backward Child and His Mother: A Psychoanalytic Study.* Pantheon Books: 1st American edition, 1972.

McGilchrist, I. (2009). *The Master and his Emissary: The Divided Brain and the Making of the Western World.* Yale University Press.

Meltzer, D. (1967). *The Psychoanalytic Process.* London: Heinemann.

Meltzer, D. (1973). Routine and inspired interpretations: their relation to the weaning process in analysis, pp. 290–306. In: *Sincerity and other Works, Collected Papers of Donald Meltzer.* Alberto Hahn (Ed.). London: Karnac, 1994.

Meltzer, D. (1975a). *Explorations in Autism. A Psycho-analytical Study.* London: The Roland Harris Educational Trust. Perthshire: Clunie Press.

Meltzer, D. (1975b). Dimensionality as a parameter of mental functioning; its relation to narcissistic organization, pp. 223–238. In: *Explorations in Autism. A Psycho-analytical Study.* London: The Roland Harris Educational Trust. Perthshire: Clunie Press.

Meltzer, D. (1976). Temperature and distance as technical dimensions of interpretation, pp. 374–386. In: *Sincerity and other Works, Collected Papers of Donald Meltzer.* Alberto Hahn (Ed.). London: Karnac, 1994.

Meltzer, D. (1984). *Dream Life. A Re-examination of the Psycho-analytical Theory and Technique.* The Roland Harris Trust Library, No. 12. Perthshire: Clunie Press.

Meltzer, D. (1986a). The psychoanalytic process: twenty years on, the setting of the analytic encounter and the gathering of the transference, pp. 551–556, In: *Sincerity and other Works, Collected Papers of Donald Meltzer.* Alberto Hahn (Ed.). London: Karnac, 1994.

Meltzer, D. (1986b). Clinical application of Bion's Concept "reversal of alpha-function", pp. 116–121. *Studies in Extended Metapsychology. Clinical Applications of Bion's Ideas.* The Roland Harris Trust Library No. 13. Perthshire: Clunie Press.

Meltzer, D. (1986c). Concerning the perception of one's own attributes and its relation to language development, pp. 175–186. *Studies in Extended Metapsychology. Clinical Applications of Bion's Ideas.* The Roland Harris Trust Library No. 13. Perthshire: Clunie Press.

Meltzer, D. (1992). *The Claustrum. An investigation of Claustrophobic* Phenomena. The Roland Harris Trust Library, No. 15. Perthshire: Clunie Press.

Meltzer, D. (1994). *Sincerity and other Works, Collected Papers of Donald Meltzer,* Alberto Hahn (Ed.). London: Karnac, 1994.

Meltzer, D., & Williams, M. H. (1988). The undiscovered country: the shape of the aesthtic conflict in Hamlet, pp. 84–133. *The Apprehension of Beauty.* The Roland Harris Trust Library, No. 14. Perthshire: Clunie Press.

Money-Kyrle, R. (1968). Cognitive development. In: *The Collected Papers of Roger Money Kyrle*. The Roland Harris Educational Trust Library, No. 7, Perthshire: Clunie Press, 1978, pp. 416–433.

Ornitz, O. M., & Ritvo, E. R. (1968). Perceptual inconstancy in early infantile autism. *Archives of General Psychiatry, 18*: 76–98.

Panofsky, E. (1927). Die Perspektive als "symbolische form". In: *Vorträge der Bibliothek Warburg 1924/1925*. Leipzig-Berlin.

Polacco, G. W. (2003). *Internal Landscapes and Foreign Bodies: Eating Disorders and Other Pathologies*. London: Karnac.

Quinton, M. (2002). *Concepts and Guidelines for Baby Treatment*. Albuquerque, New Mexico: Clinicians View.

Read, H. (1964). *A Concise History of Modern Sculpture*. London: Thames and Hudson, 1985, pp. 159–160.

Robertson, J. (2005). A psychoanalytic perspective on the work of physiotherapist with infants at risk of neurological problems. Comparing the theoretical background of physiotherapy and psychoanalysis, *International Journal of Infant Observation and its Applications, 8/3*. London: Routledge.

Schooler, L. (2003). *The Blue Bear. A Tue Story of Friendship and Discovery in the Alaskan Wild*. New York: Harper Collins, pp. 23–27.

Segal, H. (1957). Notes on symbol formation. *International Journal of Psychoanalysis, 75*: 611–618. Also in: E. B. Spillius (Ed.), *Melanie Klein Today, vol. 1: Mainly Theory*. London: Routledge, 1988.

Stern, D. N. (2010). *Forms of Vitality: Exploring Dynamic Experience in Psychology, the Arts, Psychotherapy, and Development*. Oxford: University Press.

Storaro, V. (2010). *Writing with Light*. Milano: Electa Mondadori.

Symington, N. (1981). The psychotherapy of a subnormal patient. *British Journal of Medical Psychology, 54*: 187–199.

Tagore, R. (1903). Morte del bambino. *Canto di Infanzia (Sissu)*. Marino Rigon (Ed.). Parma: Guanda, 1979, p. 142. Translated for this edition by Aldo Grassi: Oxford.

Tagore, R. (1913). The beginning. *The Crescent Moon*. London & New York: MacMillan and Company.

Tagore, R. (1916). *Fruit-Gathering*. New York: The Macmillan Company, 1916.

Trevarthen, C. (1974). Conversation with a two month old. *New Scientist, 2*: 230–235.

Trevarthen, C., & Hubley, P. (1978). Secondary intersubjectivity: confidence, confiding and acts of meaning in the first year. In: *Action Gesture and Symbol: the emergence of language*, A. Lock (ed.). London: Academic Press.

Ungaretti, G. (1888–1970). *Il Porto Sepolto—The Buried Port*, 1916 Cornell University Press, p. 228, 1975; or a new translation: *Selected Poems by*

Giuseppe Ungaretti, A Bilingual Edition. Translation, introduction, notes by Andrew Frisardi, Published April 1st 2004 by Farrar, Straus and Giroux.

Veronesi, S. (2010). *XY*. Roma: Fandango, p. 83. Translated for this edition by Aldo Grassi: Oxford.

Vianello, R. (1980 [1991]). *Ricerche psicologiche sulla religiosità infantile*. Firenze: Giunti & Barbera. Translated for this edition by Aldo Grassi: Oxford.

Waddell, M. (1998). *Inside Lives: Psychoanalysis and the Growth of the Personality*. London: Duckworth. Reprinted London: Karnac, 2002.

Williams, M. H. (2005). *The Psychoanalytic Contributions of Donald Meltzer*. A Memorial Conference, Tavistock Clinic, November 11th–12th.

Williams, M. H. (2010a). Beneficence in space: on life drawing. In: *The Aesthetic Development. The Poetic Spirit of Psychoanalysis. Essays on Bion, Meltzer, Keats*. London: Karnac, pp. 122–131.

Williams, M. H. (2010b). *The Aesthetic Development. The Poetic Spirit of Psychoanalysis. Essays on Bion, Meltzer, Keats*. London: Karnac.

Wittgenstein, L. (1953). *Philosophical Investigations*. Oxford: Blackwell, 2009.

Zehou, Li. (1988). *The Path of Beauty: A Study of Chinese Aesthetics*. Hong Kong: Oxford University Press, 1994.

INDEX